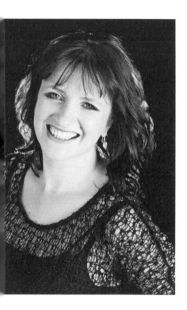

Sarah Flower, a leading nutritionist and author of many cookery books, is passionate about healthy eating and a keen advocate of the sugar-free and low-carb way of eating. She has trained with *The Real Meal Revolution*, originally set up by Professor Noakes and Jonno Proudfoot, both of whom advise banting/LCHF (low carbohydrate, high fat) and is now herself a banting coach in the UK. Sarah writes for a number of publications, including the *Daily Mail*, *Top Santé* magazine and *Healthista*. She appears regularly on BBC Radio Devon.

Also by Sarah Flower

The Busy Mum's Plan-ahead Cookbook

The Sugar-Free Family Cookbook

Eat Well, Spend Less

The Healthy Lifestyle Diet Cookbook

The Healthy Halogen Cookbook

The Healthy Slow Cooker Cookbook

Perfect Baking with Your Halogen Oven

Halogen Cooking for Two

The Everyday Halogen Family Cookbook

The Everyday Halogen Oven Cookbook

Slow Cook, Fast Food

Low-Carb Slow Cooker

Eating to Beat Type 2 Diabetes

Slow Cooker Family Classics

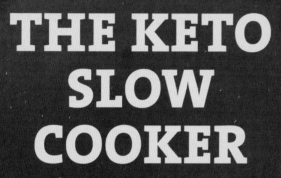

THE KETO
SLOW
COOKER

Simple, Delicious, Healthy Ketogenic

Recipes for Busy People

Sarah Flower

ROBINSON

ROBINSON

First published in Great Britain in 2020 by Robinson

1 2 3 4 5 6 7 8 9 10

A CIP catalogue record for this book
is available from the British Library.

ISBN 978-1-47214-495-9

Designed by Thextension
Typeset in The Serif & The Sans
Printed and bound in Great Britain by Bell and Bain Ltd, Glasgow

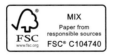

Papers used by Robinson are from well-managed forests
and other responsible sources.

Robinson
An imprint of Little, Brown Book Group
Carmelite House, 50 Victoria Embankment, London EC4Y 0DZ

An Hachette UK Company
www.hachette.co.uk

www.littlebrown.co.uk

The recommendations given in this book are solely intended
as education and should not be taken as medical advice.

Contents

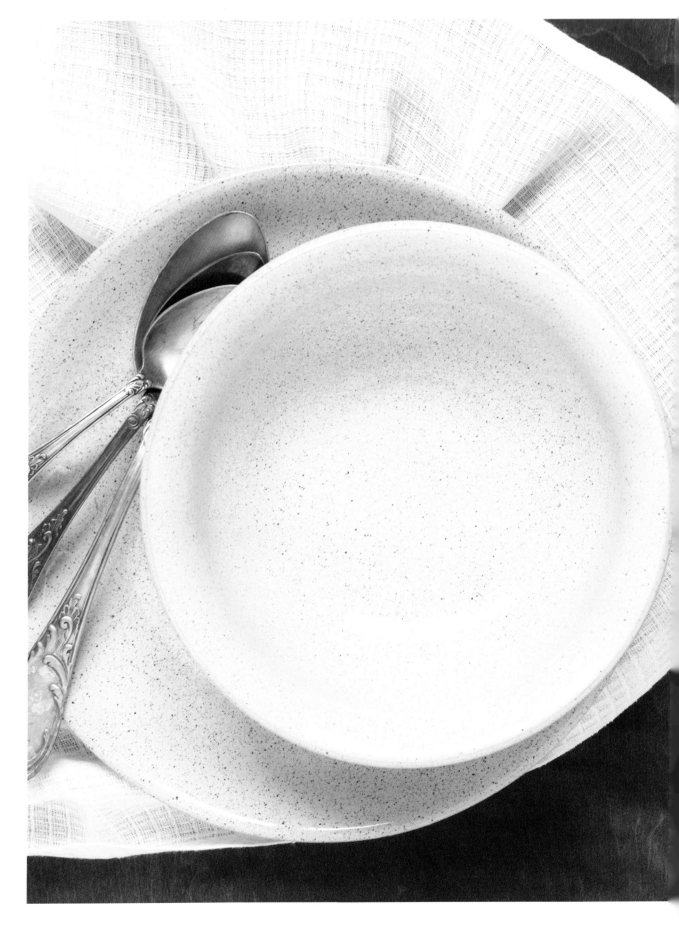

Introduction

I have been following a low-carb way of eating for around five years now. As a nutritionist, I thought I knew all there was to know about diet. Since training in the late 1990s, I had been dishing out the same low-fat, plenty-of-wholegrains, real-food mantra to my clients, and yes, it did work to a degree. But nothing has worked quite so well for such a wide variety of ills as the low-carb way of eating.

It was when my own health began to suffer that I started to question my vegetarian, wholegrain-rich diet and discovered the low-carb, ketogenic way of eating. Having spent the previous twenty-five years as a strict vegetarian, I changed my diet to a meaty, high-fat diet, and I would be lying if I said it wasn't a challenge. It took a while to shut off the niggling voice in my head every time I ate fatty meat. However, the results spoke for themselves. Soon after, my friends and family adopted the same way of eating having seen the benefits to my health. I then started to apply this to my clients and again saw some great transformations (alleviating the symptoms of IBS, migraines, polycystic ovary syndrome, to name a few), but most amazing was how it helped those with Type 2 diabetes, hypertension and obesity. I have also seen transformations with those suffering from autoimmune conditions, multiple sclerosis and fibromyalgia. I have since gone on to write several books on this topic, including *Eating to Beat Type 2 Diabetes*.

My low-carb/ketogenic journey has transformed my life and the way I work in clinic. I have met some amazing people, including the awesome Dr David Unwin, along with his wife Jen, who has been working tirelessly to change the way GPs treat diabetes in the UK. His work is incredibly inspiring, and it is down to his dedication and perseverance that we are now seeing the low-carb, ketogenic way of eating becoming more mainstream; it is now being recommended in GP surgeries across the UK. Every day I hear about success stories and research into degenerative diseases responding well to this way of eating.

I love cooking so mastering low-carb and ketogenic meals was important for me and my family, as well as to help my clients. I am a firm believer in lifestyle changes that are achievable in the long term, so being able to enjoy your favourite meals is critical for success. For this reason, I've spent a lot of time recreating family favourites to give them my low-carb, ketogenic twist.

This book uses my favourite kitchen gadget: the slow cooker. It is so easy to use and allows us to get on with our busy days without fuss. This is my second low-carb slow cooker book and I have enjoyed playing with recipes to achieve the lowest carb count without losing out on taste. Please note: all the timings and recommendations in this book are done on a new slow cooker – either my Crockpot Multi-Cooker or my Ninja Foodi. If you have an older cooker or a different model, you may want to check the temperatures as these can vary from one machine to another. Older slow cookers can have 'hot spots' where things can catch when on the high setting. If this sounds like your machine, opt for a lower setting as this can avoid potential disasters. For more information and advice do read *How to Use Your Slow Cooker* (pages 1–7).

I hope you enjoy this book. I always welcome emails from readers and would love to hear how you have got on with this book. You can also reach out to me if you have any questions on this way of eating – I am always happy to help. Please visit www.sarahflower.co.uk, where you will also find links to my Facebook groups and pages. I will also be updating new recipes and ideas on my recipe site www.everydaysugarfree.co.uk, so subscribe for regular updates. You can follow me on Twitter and Instagram @MsSarahFlower. If you have enjoyed this book, I hope you will recommend it to others.

Good luck and good health,

Sarah xx

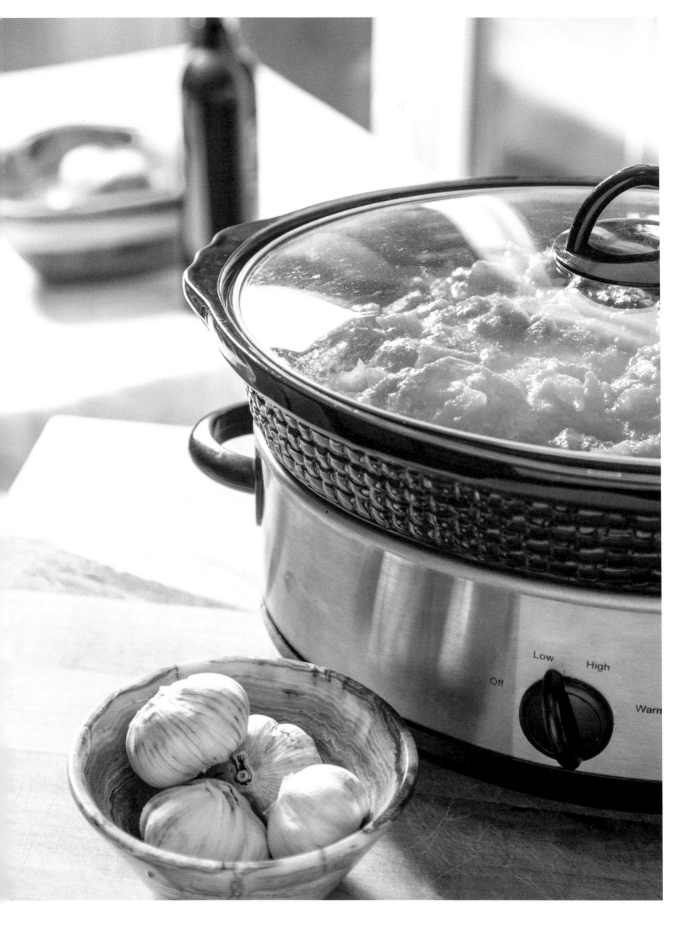

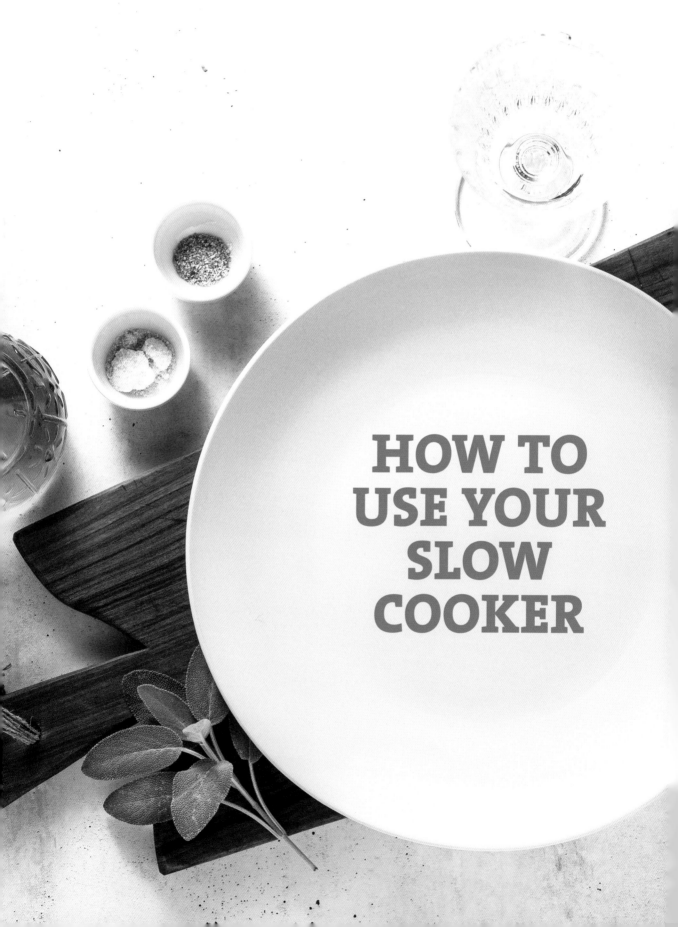

HOW TO USE YOUR SLOW COOKER

I love slow cookers…

Whether you are a slow cooker newbie or a seasoned pro, I would urge you to read this chapter in order to familiarise yourself with your machine and how to use it. Slow cookers are very popular for a good reason, but they can vary in style, use, temperature and cooking times so please remember my timings are a guide. The important factor is to get to know your machine and adapt the recipes to suit.

I love slow cookers. They are brilliant for busy people who want to come home to a wholesome meal at the end of the day, but they also maintain the nutrient value of the food. They are a great tool for saving money as you can use cheaper cuts of meat that may be tougher when cooked by traditional means, but when slow-cooked produce the most delicious, tender meat. These cuts are also much more nutrient-dense and often contain more collagen, which is great for overall health, including gut health. I make my own bone broth in the slow cooker and it is packed with nutrients and flavour. Those following a low-carb, ketogenic way of eating tend on the whole to eat more animal-based products and meat, which suits slow-cooking.

What to buy?

You can buy slow cookers from as little as £15. We are also seeing an increased popularity for multi-cookers, of which I am a huge fan (see below). When buying a slow cooker or multi-cooker, it is important to consider how it is going to be used. Think about the size of the machine. Some look quite big but the actual size of the stock pot may not be as big as you need. If you are cooking for a large family or like to plan ahead and freeze food, you may be better off spending more money and investing in a larger machine. Go to an electrical store where you can actually view the machines – even if you don't buy from them, it will give you an idea of the machines on sale and what your requirements are.

I would also strongly recommend that you buy the best you can afford. These are the functions I can't live without:

- **Multi-function** These machines are great as they combine various functions in one. The best part for me is being able to switch from sauté to slow cooker all in one machine. This is great for when you want to sauté or brown off meat prior to slow cooking as it saves time and washing up (which is a win-win for me).

- **Timer/digital display** The digital timer setting is great as it switches automatically from high or low to 'keep warm' once it has reached its set time, so no fear of overcooking and spoiling your food if you are late home.

- **Auto** Some machines have an auto button. This basically means it will start off on high and once the temperature has been reached it will switch down to low; again, perfect if you are out of the house as it means you don't have to watch over the slow cooker.

Know your own machine

This is really important! Every machine is different. If you are new to buying a machine, I would recommend buying one with a timer or digital switch as detailed above, so it can turn itself to warm once the time is reached – this saves any possible disasters with overcooking. Most models have a high and low setting.

If you have an old machine, check its temperature gauge is working correctly and also that it cooks evenly. Some can get much hotter in places, which can result in burning on the base or around the edges when left on high for long periods. If you are worried, only use it on low. The temperature should not create a boil – it should be a low, slow cook and not a fast, boiling one.

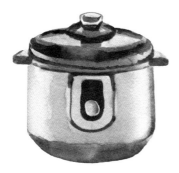

Multi-cookers

As a massive fan of the slow cooker I thought I knew all there was to know about these machines. That was until I discovered the multi-cooker. It can be used to slow-cook, sauté, bake, roast and some also have pressure cooker and even air fryer modes. Some multi-cookers have solid, pressured lids, which means you have no view of the food inside – this isn't necessarily a problem but it does mean you have to break the seal if you need to look at the food inside. I have also noticed when reviewing machines that some multi-cooker slow cooker functions – specifically the variety of settings available, the timings and cooking temperatures – can vary compared to standard slow cookers. Get to know your machine as you may have to adjust the temperature or timings to suit each recipe. I love the CrockPot Multi-Cooker as a simple multi-cooker with sauté, bake and roast function, but my absolute favourite is the Ninja Foodi as it combines all the functions, including air fryer.

To sauté or not to sauté

Recipes often tell you to sauté onions or brown the meat. I have tried with and without, and, to be honest, I really did not notice much difference in the taste, but the colour is more appealing if you sauté first and it also helps to seal the meat. If you are cooking a whole chicken, for example, remember that this will not brown, so may look a bit unappealing. Sautéing the chicken also stops it from flaking into the dish. All multi-cookers offer a sauté option and you may find that your slow cooker has a sauté function while others may come with hob-proof inserts, allowing you to transfer from one heat source to the other. You will need to refer to the manufacturer's instructions for more information. Each recipe will detail both techniques, allowing you to choose which you prefer.

Cooking techniques

All slow cookers will come with full manufacturer's instructions, recipe suggestions and even a useful helpline if you get stuck. I strongly advise you read these booklets before using your machine. Here are some reminders:

• Some cookers need to be preheated, which can take up to 15 minutes; others heat up quickly so you may not need to do this.

• The recipes will occasionally have the option of cooking on high or low, depending on how quickly you need the meal. If you are not confident with your slow cooker or suspect its temperature is hotter than it should be, always cook on low.

• As a general rule of thumb, one hour in a conventional oven is the same as 2–3 hours on high in a slow cooker or 6 hours on low.

• Some slow cookers have an auto setting – this basically means it heats up on high quickly then, when it reaches temperature, reverts to low for the remainder of the cooking time. This helps food, especially meat, reach a safe temperature quickly.

• Some machines have a warm setting. This is useful if the food has reached its maximum cooking time and you are just wanting to keep it warm. However, if you don't have a warm setting the low setting is enough (food can cook for 10 hours without starting to spoil).

• The key point to remember about slow cooking is that once you start cooking, you should avoid removing the lid as this reduces the temperature and then it takes longer for the slow cooker to get back up to the required temperature. The outer edge of the lid forms a seal – sometimes this may spit or bubble out, but this is quite normal. Only remove it when absolutely necessary – ideally just when it finishes cooking or, if necessary, in the last 30 minutes of cooking to add key ingredients. If you are the sort of person who likes to keep an eye on things, opt for a slow cooker with a glass lid (although this is not foolproof as they do get steamed up!).

• Always defrost any frozen ingredients thoroughly before placing them in the slow cooker, especially meat. The slow cooker is designed to cook safely at low temperatures but if your cooker does not maintain the required heat, it could increase the risk of food poisoning caused by the spread of bacteria. However, foods such as peas, sweetcorn, prawns and other quick-cook foods can be added frozen for the last 30 minutes of cooking time, as long as your slow cooker is set to High; otherwise they should be defrosted.

• If you plan to store meals that you have cooked in your slow cooker in your fridge or freezer, make sure they are cooled completely before placing in your containers and popping into the fridge or freezer.

• When adding liquids such as stock or water, it is better to use warm liquids (not boiling) rather than cold to maintain the temperature.

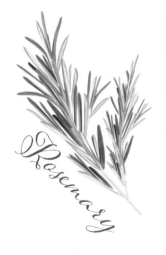

• Fresh herbs can be used, but tend to lose their intense flavours over longer cooking times. If I am using fresh herbs, I add them in the last 30 minutes of cooking or as a garnish.

• Some vegetables, especially root vegetables, take a long time to soften in the slow cooker; you can speed up the process by sautéing the vegetables prior to adding to the dish, or simply by chopping them into smaller chunks. Always place in the slow cooker first to ensure they are cooked well, making sure the vegetables are thoroughly immersed in the stock, ideally on the base as this is the hottest area.

• Be careful when adding dairy products to the slow cooker. This should be done in the last hour or so of cooking to avoid them curdling.

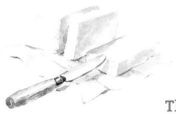

Top Tip
Xanthan gum can be hard to mix into stock. Instead, mix it with some butter and this helps it absorb into the stock, avoiding slimy clumps.

Thickening

You may need to adjust the liquid content of your dish, depending on your personal taste as well as the temperature of your slow cooker. The slow cooker does not evaporate liquid as much as other cooking methods so you may need to thicken the soups or casseroles. If you find your slow cooker does evaporate liquid, it may be overheating so check the temperature and cook on low if you are concerned. Adding more water or stock is simple and can be done at any stage. If you have added too much liquid or the meal has become too watery (sometimes this can also be due to the water content of the meat), you can thicken using xanthan gum, glucomannan fibre, coconut flour or arrowroot. Simply mix a teaspoon or two with some water to form a paste and add to the liquid; it should thicken as it heats.

Cakes

I have made keto and low-carb cakes in the slow cooker and these have been really tasty, although the texture can sometimes be different from oven-baked cakes. I think it is more about your personal taste. I have cooked cakes simply by placing the cake dish in the slow cooker and adding water to the base to create creating a bain-marie (this works well with sponge puddings and cheesecakes). If your slow cooker is large enough, you may be able to get a cake tin inside. If not, you can use a large cake liner or grease the inside well and line with baking parchment. You can also use individual ramekin dishes – if this is the case, you will need to reduce the cooking time by half. The slow cooker can sometimes get quite wet inside, especially with the condensation and steam. To prevent this from affecting your cakes or sponges, simply place a tea towel over the top of the slow cooker. Pop on the lid and push down firmly to form a good seal. This is not necessary if you are slow-cooking a pudding with a foil/parchment lid (see individual recipes for full details).

Freezing

If you want to get ahead, why not double up the recipe and freeze some? To do this, make sure you remove the dish from the slow cooker and allow it to cool thoroughly before freezing. You can buy special ziplock freezer bags for more liquid meals such as soups or casseroles. Always make sure your meals are completely defrosted before reheating.

Slow cooker prep

Some people like to get well ahead of the game and prep several meals and place these in the fridge or freezer. Advanced food prep can work well with the slow cooker. Simply bag up your solid ingredients (make sure you label them and add the date) and freeze or refrigerate until needed. If frozen, defrost before adding to the slow cooker along with the required stock.

Slow cooker liners

These are quite a new invention and can be useful in cutting down on the washing-up. They can also help prevent food sticking to the inside of the slow cooker, so are great when cooking items such as keto frittata, cheesecake or sponge pudding.

The Ketogenic Way of Eating

I love the low-carb and ketogenic way of eating. You may ask what is the main difference between the two ways of eating; the honest answer is not much, simply the amount of carbohydrates you eat per day. For a true ketogenic way of eating, you are aiming to put your body into fat-burning mode so that the body runs on fat converted to ketones rather than glucose. In order to maintain a ketogenic state (though this is not always necessary), you ideally need to consume around 20g net carbohydrates or fewer per day (this is a rough guide as everyone is different). With the low-carb way of eating (also known as low-carb high-fat [LCHF] the aim is to keep carbohydrates low, but not necessarily maintain a ketogenic state. Some schools of thought state that you are following a low-carb way of eating if you eat under 150g net carbohydrates per day; I find this hard to understand as 150g is quite a high amount of carbohydrates. In my clinic I have seen consistent weight loss, reversal of diabetes and other health issues when consuming no more than 30g carbohydrates, with only a handful of people responding well to a higher level of around 30–50g per day.

Another popular diet is the Paleolithic diet, also known as Paleo, Caveman or Stone Age diet. This way of eating resembles how are ancestors would supposedly have eaten during our hunter-gatherer phase. Paleo is similar in a lot of ways to low-carb, but it does not allow alcohol or dairy products (apart from butter) and does allow fruit, root veg and honey. Most people on the Paleo way of eating do not count carbs.

The Carnivore diet has grown in popularity and this has been shown to be a very effective diet for those with long-term ill health such as autoimmune conditions. Most start on a ketogenic, low-carb way of eating before progressing into the Carnivore diet, either to dip in and out of it, or to do for short periods of time. The carnivore way of eating involves purely animal products, though dairy is limited or even excluded for some.

Ketogenic and low-carb foods

Both ways of eating follow the simple plan of low carbohydrates, moderate amounts of protein and high fat. Dairy, meat, eggs and fish are your staple foods along with non-starchy vegetables and small amounts of low-fructose fruit such as berries. Remember, this diet is very strict in prohibiting processed foods, sugary foods, grains, beans and pulses, inflammatory oils and dried fruit. I have included an extensive food list in the back of the book for easy reference, but the following is a simplified version.

You can eat the following:

- All naturally cured meat, fish and poultry
- Eggs
- All dairy, though it must be in natural state, for example whole milk, full-fat yoghurt, cream, cheese, etc.
- Greens, salads, non-starchy vegetables (see page 184 for more information)
- Low-fructose berries
- Nuts and seeds (avoid cashews as they have a high carb content – see page 183 for more information)
- Chocolate (at least 85% cocoa solids), unsweetened cocoa and cacao
- Homemade bone, meat and vegetable broths

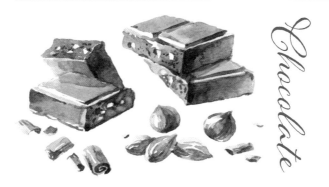

Chocolate

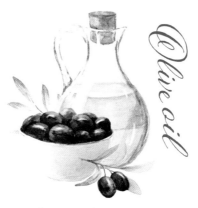

Olive oil

- Only natural oils and fats, such as coconut oil, good-quality olive oil, butter, duck fat, goose fat, ghee, pure avocado oil and pure macadamia oil
- Homemade mayonnaise and salad dressings
- Homemade or sugar-free ketchup
- All herbs and spices (as long as they do not contain sugar or wheat)
- Grain-free flours and thickeners, such as coconut flour, almond flour, ground almonds, nut and seed flour, milled seeds, xanthan gum, whey powder, arrowroot and baking powder
- Natural sweeteners, such as stevia, monk fruit, erythritol
- Coffee, tea, water

At first glance these lists may look restrictive, but please believe me when I tell you that this is far from the case. Yes, you are no longer able to have processed and junk foods, but in its place is real honest food that not only balances your blood sugars but can also reduce excess weight and improve your overall health.

I have followed this way of eating for several years now. My diet consists of a wide range of foods but is very traditional and family orientated. I can honestly say I don't miss much from my previous high-carb, low-fat vegetarian lifestyle. If I am honest, the only thing I have really missed is crisps, which I think is more to do with the salt craving coupled with the 'crunch' that is missing from the LCHF diet; to counteract this I always make sure I have some salted nuts in my cupboard, plus there are so many other lovely things to snack on, such as Parmesan, salami, kale and baked cheese crisps. I also make delicious crackers that are really crisp so give me the crunch I have missed. I could add pork scratchings, biltong or jerky, but I'm personally not a huge fan of the taste. There are lots of recipes available online if you search keto or low-carb.

Counting carbs

As I touched on at the start of this chapter, to follow the ketogenic way of eating you have to count your carbohydrates as the recommended daily amount is around 20g or less of net carbohydrates (higher if you are not worried about being in ketosis). All the recipes in this book show net carbohydrates in the nutritional information, as do all food labels in the UK. The USA differs in food labelling and nutritional calculations as food products sold there show gross carbohydrate, requiring you to deduct the fibre in order to get the net carbohydrate amount. This can cause confusion on social media forums where people are taking advice but are not aware of the differences in locations. Do not make the mistake of deducting fibre from the net carbohydrate value or you will be inadvertently underestimating the carbohydrates you are consuming.

Dairy-free

Some of you may be following a dairy-free ketogenic lifestyle. This is increasingly popular and has been shown to be very effective for those who have inflammatory and autoimmune conditions as well as stubborn weight loss. It is often one of the first things I try if a client is failing to make progress. I have included dairy-free options in many recipes. These swaps can be quite simple, such as using coconut cream instead of dairy cream. Giving up cheese can be difficult for some, but it is surprising how quickly you can adapt to a diet without dairy. I have indicated which recipes are naturally dairy free and, where applicable, I have added a note to the recipes when an ingredient can be swapped to make it dairy-free

Get swapping!

I find my clients have better results and can adapt easier to any dietary changes when I spend time helping them adapt their favourite recipes to suit the diet. It also helps when you have family members who are following a traditional high-carbohydrate diet and you want to eat similar foods. For this reason I have included a chapter of keto accompaniments and side dishes that everyone can enjoy. The following family favourites are very easy to switch to low-carb.

TRADITIONAL RECIPE	LCHF SWAP
Spaghetti bolognese	Switch spaghetti for spiralized courgette
Curry with rice	Switch rice for broccoli or cauliflower rice
Roast dinner	Avoid potatoes but fill up on extra low-carb veggies and meat. I make celeriac roast potatoes and low-carb Yorkshire puddings.
Pizza	There are lots of LCHF and keto pizza recipes, including pizzas with cauliflower and courgette bases.
Burgers	You can make some amazing keto and low-carb grain-free bread recipes, or simply ditch the bun and have extra salad.
Chilli con carne	Leave out the red kidney beans and serve with broccoli or cauliflower rice. You can also make tacos from grated Parmesan.
Lasagne	Swap pasta sheets for strips of courgette, aubergine, butternut squash or even bacon.
Mashed potato	Cauliflower or celeriac mash made with lots of cheese and butter is amazing! Use as a topping for shepherd's pie or serve with a hearty casserole.
Breaded items, such as chicken nuggets, fish fingers, Scotch eggs etc.	Use ground pork scratchings combined with Parmesan to make a crunchy coating; simply dip food into a beaten egg, then dip into the ground scratchings and bake as normal.

Bread	There are numerous recipes for keto bread online. Some use psyllium husk powder, readily available from health food shops or online, however, some brands can turn your bread a purple colour!
Cakes and biscuits	The keto way of eating is all about home-cooked produce so don't expect to walk into a supermarket and buy keto-friendly ready-made food. My previous books, *Eating to Beat Type 2 Diabetes*, *The Sugar-Free Family Cookbook* and my website www.everydaysugarfree.co.uk contain lots of keto cakes, biscuit and dessert recipes to satisfy the sweetest tooth.
Breakfast cereals	Most cereals are poor in nutrients and full of sugar so swap for a healthier breakfast with eggs, a cooked breakfast or some keto granola.

Quick snack ideas

This is a simple reference guide to the quick and easy snacks you should stock up on – ideal for when you are hungry or if you want to take something with you to work or for a day out.

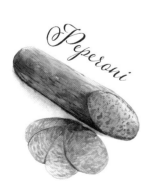

- Hard-boiled eggs
- Nuts and seeds (not cashews)
- Dark chocolate (at least 85% cocoa solids)
- Cheese
- Pepperoni, salami, Parma ham and prosciutto
- Antipasti platters
- Biltong and jerky
- Salads

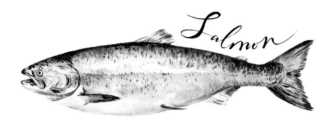

- Olives
- Fish, including salmon and tuna
- All meat
- Cream or yoghurt with berries
- Nut butter with vegetable sticks
- Parmesan crisps
- Pork scratchings

Golden rules

• Plan, plan and plan again. Writing shopping lists and meal plans really does help, especially in the first few weeks of eating this way. You don't want to come home from work and have nothing to eat – that is a sure-fire way to end up eating the wrong food.

• Always read the labels and keep an eye out for added sugar (see page 00). This diet is all about eating real food in its natural state.

• Don't fear the fat. We need to embrace our fat, so fill up on healthy fats found in oily fish, avocados and nuts. Buy good-quality meat and eat the fat. All dairy products must be full-fat versions.

• This diet is high in fat, with moderate amounts of protein and very low carbs. Your body is incredibly clever and has the ability to create more carbohydrates and glucose from protein, so you do need to keep protein in moderation.

• Any change in diet can result in a change in bowel habits. A high-carb diet can produce very messy, sticky poos. This way of eating creates firmer, cleaner poos, but the transition may result in constipation. The best way to make sure your bowels are in tip-top condition is to add a daily dose of bowel flora in the form of a probiotic. Always choose the best quality you can afford and I would strongly advise you to avoid 'yoghurt' drinks as often the healthy bacteria fail to reach the large intestine. Also, a high dose of vitamin C (in the form of a supplement) can really help get things moving, as can magnesium in citrate form. You must also drink plenty of water every day. Some of my clients find relief by taking a psyllium husk capsule daily.

• You can still make cakes, biscuits and desserts and maintain the ketogenic way of eating. I like to do this as I feel it makes this way of life more sustainable over the long term and reduces the feeling that you are missing out or losing the joy of food. I recommend using stevia, erythritol or monk fruit sweeteners as these are very low in carbs and have very little impact on your blood sugars. However some people find that sweet foods only perpetuate their cravings so you may prefer to avoid them all together.

• Only eat when you are hungry. Many of us have got into the habit of snacking throughout the day, which continually stimulates an insulin response. I have got into the habit of eating just two meals a day, with the second meal normally fairly light, and I am rarely hungry. As you consume more fat, you will feel more satisfied, the cravings will diminish, and you will stay fuller for longer.

• Think about fruit in a different way. See it as nature's candy, full of sugar, so to be eaten only occasionally. Berries have the lowest sugar content so are the best choice. As long as you eat a good balanced diet, with plenty of vegetables packed with antioxidants and phytonutrients, you will not go without.

• The keto way of eating is totally grain-free. That may seem daunting at first, but it is really quite simple. Most of my clients see a dramatic difference in their health from avoiding grains, including less bloating, IBS, inflammation and headaches. Some fail to realise the benefits until they have a grain-based meal and immediately start to feel unwell.

The Keto Store Cupboard

This is a rough guide to what you need to stock up on when you embark on a ketogenic lifestyle and is based on what I use myself. I try to use everyday foods, so this list is quite basic. Remember: you are not stocking up on lots of processed foods, but making your own – even condiments.

Natural sweeteners

Some people like to use natural sweeteners, especially if they follow a low-carb way of eating rather than the stricter ketogenic diet. Others find it increases their desire for sweet food so prefer to leave them alone. I have been on a low-carb diet for a number of years and I do enjoy some sweet foods, but I don't eat a huge amount as my palate has changed significantly over the years. I used to be a complete sweetaholic, loving cakes, desserts and confectionery and I am sure if I started eating sugar again, I would very quickly return to these old habits. Fortunately, natural sweeteners don't have the same effect on me, which is good as natural sweeteners shouldn't be an excuse to eat loads of sweet foods. They are a tool to help you in the transition phase to reduce your sugar cravings. The further down the sugar-free road you go, the less you will crave sweet food. You will also find you can dramatically reduce the quantity of natural sweeteners in your recipes as your palate changes. Here are some natural sweeteners to look out for:

Erythritol blend This sugar alcohol is found in grapes and pears. Erythritol contains zero calories and does not affect blood sugar or insulin levels during or after consumption, making it safe for diabetics and for those following a low-carb diet. Unlike other sugar alcohols, such as xylitol, erythritol is well absorbed from the digestive tract, passes into the urine and is eliminated from the body, so it does not have a laxative side effect. I use Sukrin products, but you can also use Natvia and PureVia brands, available in UK supermarkets. Swerve is also very popular in the US and is becoming more widely available (online) here in the UK. You can also buy icing sugar products within most of these ranges.

Sukrin Gold Made with erythritol, this is a great alternative to brown sugar; I use it quite a lot to create a deep, sweet flavour. I also use Sukrin Fibre Syrup, which, although expensive, does go a long way and is great for creating chewy nut bars and granola, or simply to drizzle over a keto porridge in the winter months.

Monk fruit This is the relatively new kid on the block. It is very sweet (around 150 times sweeter than sugar), but not as sweet as stevia. It is a fruit grown on a vine, native to South East Asia. You can buy it in granule form.

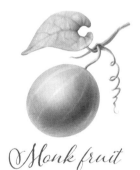

Monk fruit

Stevia Stevia is a subtropical wild plant. Its leaves contain glycosides, whose sweetening power is between 250 and 400 times their equivalent in sugar. Stevia contains no calories and no carbohydrates. It does not raise blood sugar or stimulate an insulin response, so, for many, it is the preferred choice, as it is completely natural. Stevia is very sweet and the cheapest natural sweetener out of all three, but it does have a strange aftertaste, which is hard to control and depends on the brand you use and your personal taste. I use Sweetleaf Stevia drops – they are very good and have the least aftertaste. Always check the label to ensure it is pure stevia and not a blend of stevia with sugar.

Xylitol This is a natural sugar alternative first discovered in birch wood. It has now been found in a host of other plants and fruits, such as sweetcorn and plums. Xylitol looks and tastes just like normal granulated sugar. It can, however, have a laxative effect in some people if eaten to excess. You also need to keep xylitol, or any food made with it, away from dogs as it can be very dangerous for them, even in small amounts. In the UK the most popular brand available in supermarkets is Total Sweet. Xylitol does cause a spike in blood sugars, so it is not as good for the ketogenic way of eating as erythritol, monk fruit or stevia.

Common misconceptions about natural sweeteners

You will find lots of 'natural' sweeteners in food, some claiming to be sugar-free, but I tend to stick to stevia, erythritol and monk fruit. Food manufacturers and many food bloggers have recognised the need to reduce sugar but are focusing on refined sugar. However, our bodies don't differentiate between refined or unrefined sugars. Honey, molasses, maple syrup, dates, coconut sugar and agave syrup are all sugars, and they spike blood sugar levels, and therefore an insulin response, as well as delivering high levels of fructose so they cannot be part of the ketogenic way of eating.

We are also seeing a rise in 'sugar-free' products in supermarkets. I am a member of lots of ketogenic and low-carb forums and it never fails to amaze me how people bend the rules and offer dodgy advice to newbies. I have seen people suggest wheat products as part of a ketogenic lifestyle as well as heavily processed foods. People also get very excited about sugar-free sweets, chocolate and snacks, but these can contain some less-than-ideal natural sweeteners.

• Sucralose is often found in products claiming to be low-carb or sugar-free but it does spike blood sugar levels moderately in a similar way to xylitol. Unlike xylitol, sucralose is an artificial sweetener and has been linked to health issues including changes in the gut flora, weight gain, nausea, bloating, muscle pain and inflammation.

• Dextrose is made from corn and is very similar to glucose. It does spike blood sugars moderately but is also associated to bloating, swelling, blood clots, inflammation and gut issues.

• Maltitol is a sugar alcohol often found in sugar-free confectionery and chocolate products. Some people can tolerate this; however, I find it can have a laxative effect as well as increase stomach cramps and flatulence. It also can increase blood sugars.

- Mannitol and sorbitol are also sugar alcohols and, once again, they can cause stomach upsets including diarrhoea.

- Inulin is part of the fructans family. It is an indigestible fibre but it can cause fermentation in the gut, leading to diarrhoea, flatulence and bloating. Some people can tolerate small amounts.

Artificial sweeteners

I avoid these completely as I have read too many studies linking their use to mental health problems and health complaints. There is now mounting evidence to show that artificial sweeteners are highly addictive and can increase your sugar cravings. They can also contribute to insulin resistance and diabetes and have been linked to headaches, cancer, hypertension, impaired gut health, organ damage, anxiety and even seizures.

The well-stocked keto kitchen

Making sure that your cupboards, fridge and freezer are stocked with the right ingredients will make switching to the ketogenic lifestyle much easier. Here are my essential ingredients.

Store cupboard

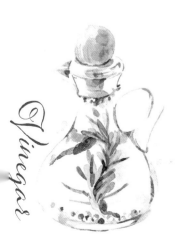

Almond or coconut flour Cake recipes often call for almond flour or coconut flour. Almond flour is quite expensive so I often use ground almonds. Coconut flour is a great flour alternative; it absorbs up to ten times its volume so you may need to add more liquid when you are using this flour. A good 'all-purpose' flour is three parts almond flour or ground almonds to one part coconut flour.

Apple cider vinegar I like to drink this every day as it has some amazing health benefits. I also add this when making bone broth as it helps pull out the nutrients. You can use this in place of white wine vinegar in salad dressings.

Cocoa/cacao It's a case of personal preference whether you prefer cocoa or cacao. Look for unsweetened cocoa.

Dark chocolate You can buy good-quality dark chocolate but always check the carb content. Choose chocolate that is at least 85% cocoa solids; there are 100% cocoa solids available but if you are a newbie you may want to ease yourself into the strong taste of dark chocolate. If you are buying dark chocolate chips do check the carb content as many supermarket varieties only contain about 50% cocoa. Go to a health food shop or look online for better options.

Coconut I have shredded coconut as well as desiccated coconut. I use the shredded coconut in my granola and nut bars.

Coconut oil Absolutely essential as it is used a lot in ketogenic recipes.

Chia seeds These little seeds are packed with goodness. They are great to use as a thickener and they make wonderful porridge and creamy desserts.

Gelatine I use gelatine powder by Great Lakes as I like the grass-fed, natural variety but you can use sheets if you prefer.

Nuts I use a lot of nuts, mostly almonds, pecans, walnuts, hazelnuts, macadamia and Brazil nuts. I also use fresh nuts and blend them to make nut butters and nut flours. Store unused nut flours in the freezer to prevent them going rancid. Nuts are also great to make your own granola and nut bars. You can also make spicy nuts as a healthy replacement to crisps.

Seasonings I use a lot of seasonings and make my own blends. It is best if you can buy these in bulk as it will save money. I store them in small jars.

Seeds I have a range of seeds in my cupboard – flaxseeds, sesame seeds, pumpkin and sunflower seeds are the ones I use every day. I often sauté some seeds in coconut oil and add these to my salads to make a nice crunch and add additional nutrients. I also use seeds in homemade bread and crackers and sprinkle them on top of yoghurt.

Sun-dried tomatoes in oil I love the flavour of sun-dried tomatoes, but check the labels as some brands contain added sugar. I always keep a jar to add to food or to turn into paste. Use sparingly as unsweetened sun-dried tomatoes can be quite high in carbohydrates (12–17g per 100g).

Tinned tomatoes You can always whip up a tasty dish if you have some tinned tomatoes. I always buy the best quality I can as I find the taste far nicer. These contain around 3–4g carbohydrates per 100g.

Whey powder Although I have not used any in this recipe book, I do use organic grass-fed whey powder to make grain-free bread; it is also useful in some grain-free cake recipes. I occasionally add it to smoothies.

Xanthan gum Use this as a thickener – simply sprinkle on to your dish and stir well.

Yeast extract I use this in my cooking as it can add a good flavour. Check that your brand is sugar-free.

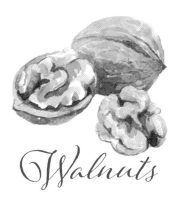

Walnuts

Fridge

Bacon I don't eat a lot of bacon but it is always good to have in the fridge. I buy good-quality bacon, free from nitrates and sugars. I bake it until it is very crispy before chopping into small pieces to add to a salad. I also use it in my main meals and, obviously, for breakfast. Buy from your local butcher; this way it shouldn't cost much more than the supermarket but will be far superior in quality.

Berries For me, fresh berries are a must-have when in season, although I only use a small handful at a time (see also frozen berries).

Butter Another essential – the low-carb and ketogenic way of eating is all about eating real food and that includes ditching all the man-made industrialised oils and margarines.

Carbonated sparkling water Controversial, I know, as some people believe it stops you absorbing nutrients. For me, it is a refreshing drink to have occasionally with slices of lemon and lime and can be good if you are withdrawing from fizzy drinks.

Cheese I always have full-fat cream cheese in my fridge as I use it for puddings, pizza bases and even cakes as it is a great binder. I keep a variety of cheeses, including extra-mature Cheddar, Brie, halloumi, Stilton and feta.

Cream I buy extra-thick cream for puddings. I also have double cream to make sauces and to add to dishes. Cream is also essential for making your own ice cream.

Eggs These are absolutely vital! I probably get through at least 24 eggs a week. All eggs used in the recipes are medium, unless otherwise stated.

Extra-virgin olive oil I buy my olive oil in tins and keep it in a cool, dark cupboard as heat, light and oxygen can destroy the nutrients and turn it rancid. My favourite brand is Pomora, a subscription-based company which offers high-quality olive oils with different natural flavour enhancers.

Mayonnaise I always have a jar of homemade mayonnaise in my fridge.

Meat and fish I buy free-range, organic chicken. We are fortunate that our beef in the UK is grass-fed, so I buy organic beef from the supermarket or rely on the local recommendations from my butcher. I also eat pork, lamb and venison. I eat steaks with salads and also like to roast a gammon joint, using the cold meat in savoury snacks and omelettes. I buy gluten-free, high-quality sausages from my butcher. I buy fresh fish but also have some tuna steaks and salmon fillets in the freezer.

Milk I use full-fat milk in my cooking but use milk sparingly as the carbohydrates can soon add up, especially if you are a fan of milky drinks or lattes! You may want to consider swapping your milky coffee for a bulletproof coffee or coffee with cream.

Vegetables and salads My fridge is always full of salads and vegetables, including avocados – a must-have! Don't let your avocados go off as you can freeze them in chunks or slices – frozen avocado is great to use in smoothies, guacamole and chocolate pudding.

Yoghurt I only buy full-fat Greek yoghurt and add my own berries and chopped nuts. I also really love plant-based coconut yoghurt (my favourite brand is The Coconut Collaborative) as it makes a refreshing change when I am a little fed up with cream.

Milk

Freezer

Berries These are a great cost-effective option when fresh berries aren't in season.

Meat and fish I never buy frozen meat but I do have chicken breasts, lardons, mince and steak in my freezer. To my shame, this is often because I don't get around to eating it in time so pop it in the freezer for another time! I usually have salmon fillets and tuna steaks in the freezer as well.

Vegetables I always have frozen peas in my freezer. Some supermarkets are now selling frozen cauliflower and broccoli rice but you can make your own so easily; I often whizz up uncooked cauliflower florets (perhaps if I've used it in a recipe and have some left over) and pop this into small bags and place in the freezer.

Bones I buy a large bag of bones (about 4kg) from my butcher for about £2 a bag. This lasts me months. I slow-cook and then store the bone broth in the freezer in small freezer bag portions. I also freeze some in ice-cube trays to pop out whenever I need to add a touch of stock to a dish.

Homemade ready-prepared meals I try to keep a range of homemade meals in my freezer for those days when I haven't got time to put something together. Always remember to label and date anything that goes in, or it can be in there for months!

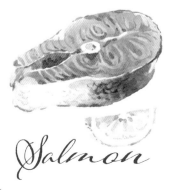

Salmon

Conversion charts and symbols

Weight

METRIC	IMPERIAL
25g	1oz
50g	2oz
75g	3oz
100g	4oz
150g	5oz
175g	6oz
200g	7oz
225g	8oz
250g	9oz
300g	10oz
350g	12oz
400g	14oz
450g	1lb

Measurements

METRIC	IMPERIAL
5cm	2in
10cm	4in
13cm	5in
15cm	6in
18cm	7in
20cm	8in
25cm	10in
30cm	12in

Liquids

METRIC	IMPERIAL	US CUP
5ml	1 tsp	1 tsp
15ml	1 tbsp	1 tbsp
50ml	2fl oz	3 tbsp
60ml	2½fl oz	¼ cup
75ml	3fl oz	⅓ cup
100ml	4fl oz	scant ½ cup
125ml	4fh oz	½ cup
150ml	5fl oz	⅔ cup
200ml	7fl oz	scant 1 cup
250ml	9fl oz	1 cup
300ml	½ pint	1¼ cups
350ml	12fl oz	1⅓ cups
400ml	¾ pint	1¾ cups
500ml	17fl oz	2 cups
600ml	1 pt	2½ cups

❄ Double up and freeze

Suitable for vegetarians

Suitable for vegans

Dairy free option

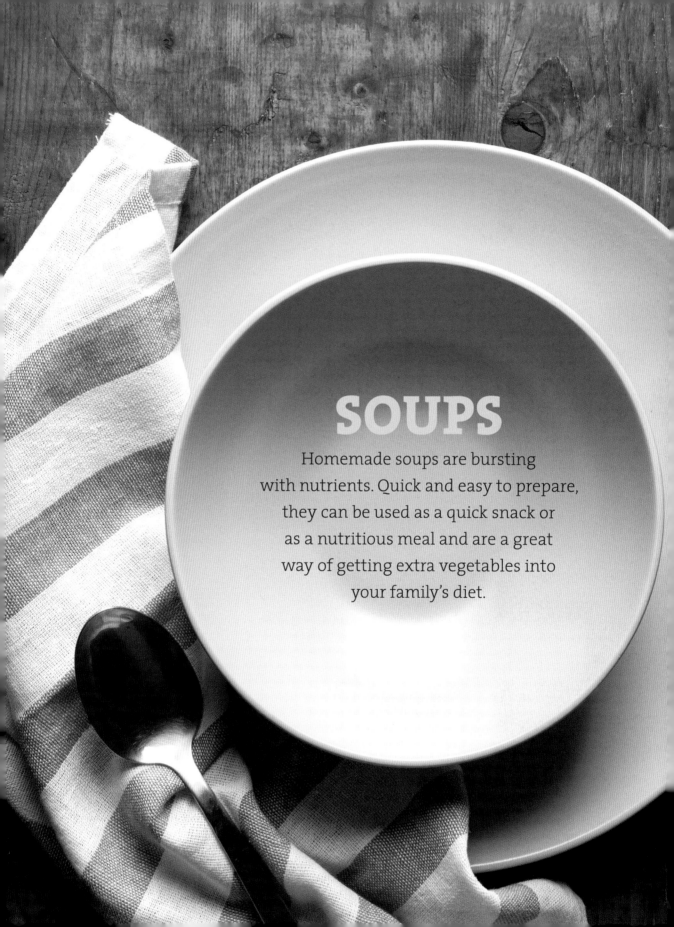

SOUPS

Homemade soups are bursting
with nutrients. Quick and easy to prepare,
they can be used as a quick snack or
as a nutritious meal and are a great
way of getting extra vegetables into
your family's diet.

They are also cheap to make and very filling. Best of all, as they are slow-cooked at a low temperature, the nutrients are maintained making the soup ultra-healthy. If you or your child has a packed lunch, consider buying a small flask and filling it with your homemade soup – perfect to fill up and warm the body during the winter months. Most soups can be frozen so fill your freezer with individual portions.

SOUP-MAKING TIPS

Stock Stock cubes can be quite overpowering and also high in salt and sugar but there are some great products available that give a more natural flavour. Try to make your own broth as it is packed with nutrients, particularly if you use animal bones. I am a huge fan of bone broth as it is packed with nutrients (see page 162). It freezes well so make a large batch and freeze in portions.

Puréeing Some people like a chunky soup, others like a smooth soup. It is purely down to personal taste. I use an electric hand blender (or stick blender) to purée my soups – they are simple to use but make sure the end of the blender is fully submerged in the soup or you will end up with it everywhere! For a really fine soup, you can then pass it through a sieve. Some chunky soups may benefit from a thicker liquid; simply remove about a quarter of the soup, purée it, then return to the soup.

Thickening soups You may need to adjust the liquid content of your soup as the slow cooker does not evaporate liquid as much as other cooking methods. Here are my top tips to thicken soups or casseroles

- Remove the lid of the slow cooker and allow the steam to evaporate until you achieve the desired thickness.
- Mix xanthan gum with butter before popping into the slow cooker.
- Mix coconut flour, glucomannan fibre or almond flour with a few tablespoons of water. Place the thickener into the slow cooker, ensuring it is evenly distributed. Turn the temperature to high and cook for 15–30 minutes until thick.

Creams Creams, milk, Greek yoghurt and crème fraîche can sometimes separate when cooked in a slow cooker for long periods so it is best to add these to soups just before serving.

Celeriac is a wonderful, versatile vegetable for the low-carber. It has a wonderful flavour, almost like a combination of celery, parsnip and potato. This soup is thick and creamy and works brilliantly with the smoky saltiness of the bacon.

Celeriac and Bacon Soup

Serves 6

❄ Ⓘ

Nutritional information per serving
404 Kcals
36g fat
5.3g net carbohydrates
13g protein

Ingredients
8 rashers of thick smoked back bacon, diced

30g butter

1 onion, finely chopped

2 garlic cloves, crushed

600g celeriac, peeled and diced

2 tsp dried thyme

1 tsp dried marjoram

1 tsp onion powder

800ml hot bone or chicken broth

250ml double cream (or use coconut cream if dairy-free)

salt and black pepper, to taste

Preheat your slow cooker, following the manufacturer's instructions.

If your slow cooker has a sauté function, switch to this before adding the bacon; if not, use a sauté pan on your hob.

Cook the bacon for 5 minutes, then remove two-thirds of it and continue to cook the remaining bacon until crispy. Place the crispy bacon on to a plate lined with kitchen towel to absorb any fat and keep to one side, ready to use as a garnish.

Place the remaining bacon back into the slow cooker, keeping it on the sauté function (or return to the sauté pan) and add the butter, onion, garlic and celeriac and cook for another 5 minutes before switching to the slow cooker function. Add the herbs, onion powder and hot broth to the slow cooker, set to Low and cook for 6–7 hours until soft.

Whizz with a stick blender until you have a smooth soup. If you don't have a stick blender, remove from slow cooker and liquidise until smooth. Stir in the cream. Cook on High for a further 15 minutes to heat through.

Season to taste and serve immediately, garnished with the crispy bacon.

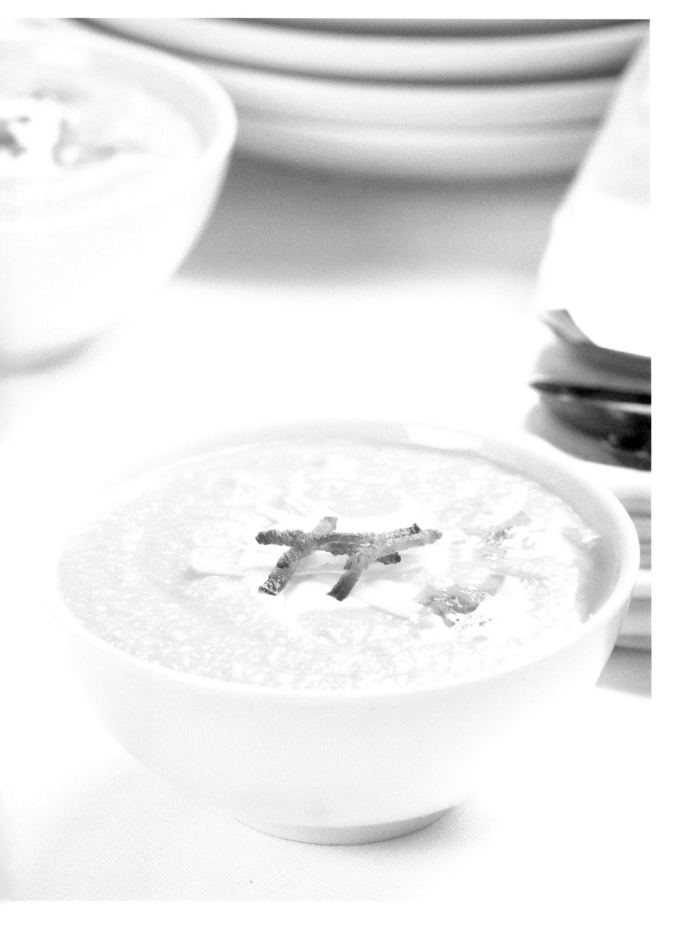

This is a very filling meal, perfect when you are looking for a winter warmer that satisfies. I love the flavour of paprika and chilli, it works so well with beef. If you don't like it hot, you can always leave out the chilli. Remember to chop your beef into small dice for this soup – any bigger and you are into casserole territory!

Fiery Beef Goulash Soup

Serves 4
❄ ⊘

Nutritional information per serving
248 Kcals
6.4g fat
10g net carbohydrates
34g protein

Ingredients
500g braising steak, diced

1 red onion, diced

3 garlic cloves, crushed

1–2 chillies, deseeded and finely chopped

1 tbsp caraway seeds, crushed

1 tsp dried marjoram

1 tbsp sweet paprika

2 tsp smoked paprika

1 tbsp tomato purée

1 large red pepper, deseeded and diced

500ml hot bone or beef broth

salt and black pepper, to taste

sour cream, to serve

Preheat your slow cooker, following the manufacturer's instructions.

Put all the ingredients except for the sour cream into your slow cooker and stir well to combine.

Set to Low and cook for 5–6 hours.

Season to taste before serving with a generous dollop of sour cream.

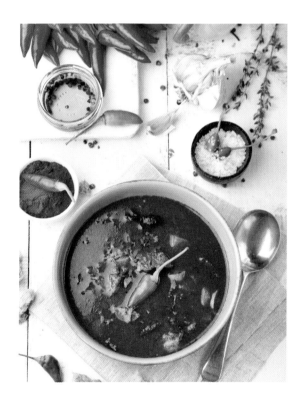

This is a hearty, spicy soup, perfect for the winter months when you want something filling and warming. It is delicious on its own, served with some keto bread or crackers, but you can also increase the fat content by topping with some chopped avocado or some strong grated cheese.

Mexican Beef Soup

Serves 4

Nutritional
information per
serving
222 Kcals
7.5g fat
9.9g net carbohydrates
25g protein

Ingredients
2 tsp coconut oil or ghee

250g stewing beef,
cut into small chunks

1 small red onion, finely
chopped

2 chillies, finely chopped

3 garlic cloves, finely
chopped

1 red pepper, deseeded
and finely chopped

1 carrot, diced

2 tbsp tomato purée

1 tbsp smoked paprika

½ tsp dried coriander

2 tsp dried oregano

500ml hot bone, chicken
or vegetable broth

salt and black pepper,
to taste

Preheat your slow cooker, following the manufacturer's instructions.

If your slow cooker has a sauté option, use this; if not, use a sauté pan on your hob. Heat the coconut oil or ghee, add the beef and cook until browned, sealing in the flavour. Place in the slow cooker (if you used a separate pan).

Add all the remaining ingredients, set to Low and cook for 6–7 hours.

Season to taste, then serve with some keto bread or crackers. If you are not dairy-free, you can finish with a sprinkle of strong grated Cheddar.

Note
if you want to reduce
the carbs even more,
leave out the carrot and
halve the tomato purée,
cutting the net carbs to
6.9g per serving.

This is a lovely, creamy soup, packed with nutrients. If I don't have broccoli, I will sometimes replace it with some kale or spinach. This is delicious with some keto bread, toasted and spread with lots of butter.

Courgette, Broccoli and Feta Soup

Serves 4
❄

Nutritional information per serving
161 Kcals
7.3g fat
6.8g net carbohydrates
14g protein

Ingredients
750g courgettes, thickly sliced

1 head of broccoli, cut into florets

2 garlic cloves, crushed

500ml hot bone or vegetable broth

100g feta cheese, crumbled

a small handful of fresh mint, chopped

Preheat your slow cooker, following the manufacturer's instructions.

Put the courgettes, broccoli, garlic and hot broth into the slow cooker. Set to Low and cook for 4–5 hours (or cook on High for 1½–2 hours if you prefer).

Fifteen minutes before serving add the feta cheese and fresh mint. Stir well and turn to High. Cook for 15 minutes before using a stick blender to blitz until smooth.

Finish with a swirl of double cream, and serve with some toasted keto bread.

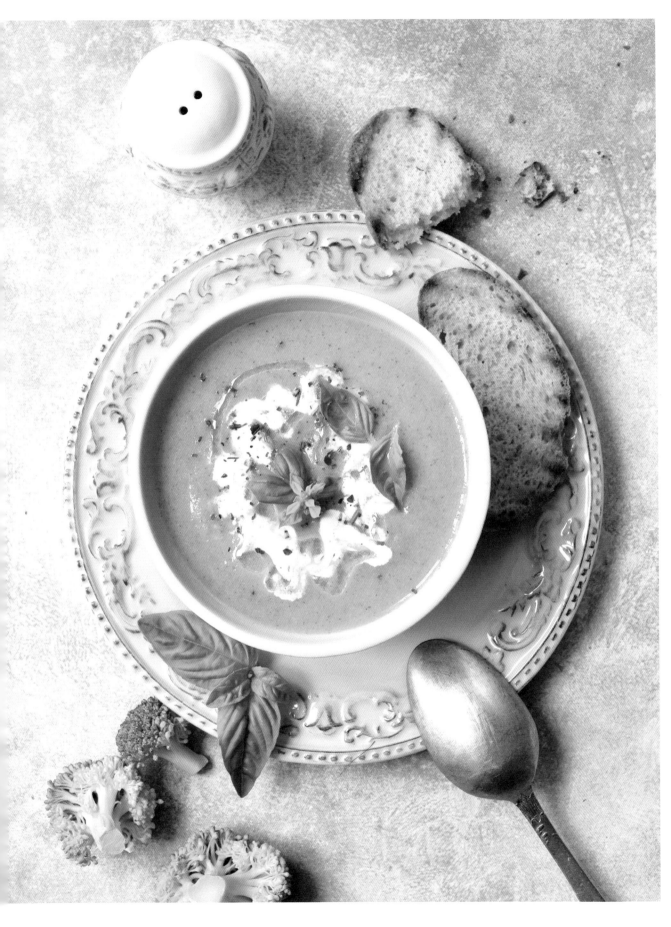

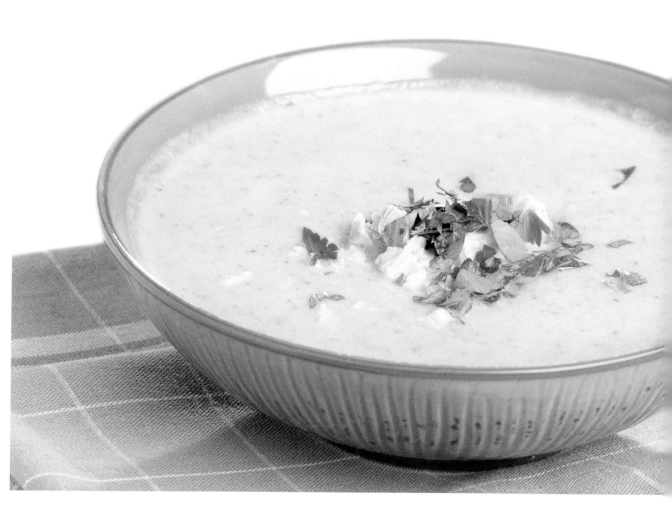

There is nothing nicer than a bowl of creamy chicken soup when you are feeling a little under par or are in need of a comforting, warming meal. This recipe uses raw chicken, but if you have leftovers you can use cooked chicken instead. If opting for cooked chicken, you can reduce the cooking time by 1–2 hours.

Creamy Chicken Soup

Serves 4
❄ Ⓓ

Nutritional information per serving
520 Kcals
40g fat
5g net carbohydrates
34g protein

Ingredients
1 onion, diced

2 celery sticks, diced

1 garlic clove, crushed

500g boneless chicken (breast or thigh), diced

500ml hot bone or chicken broth

2 tsp dried thyme

1 tsp dried parsley

300ml double cream (or use coconut cream if dairy-free)

1 tsp xanthan gum (optional)

salt and black pepper, to taste

Preheat your slow cooker, following the manufacturer's instructions.

Put all the ingredients apart from the cream and xanthan gum into the slow cooker.

Set to Low and cook for 4–5 hours.

Fifteen minutes before serving, add the double cream. If the soup needs thickening, sprinkle over the xanthan gum too. Immediately use a stick blender to blitz the soup until creamy. Set to High and allow to cook for the remaining 15 minutes.

Season to taste and serve with some keto bread or crackers.

This is an absolute classic and one of my favourites. Traditionally this is made with potato, which adds creaminess due to the starch content; however, it works really well with celeriac.

Creamy Broccoli and Stilton Soup

Serves 4
❄

Nutritional information per serving
285 Kcals
19g fat
6.2g net carbohydrates
19g protein

Ingredients
1 onion, finely chopped
100g celeriac, peeled and diced
1 large head of broccoli, cut into florets
650ml hot bone, chicken or vegetable broth
200g Stilton or other blue cheese, crumbled
salt and black pepper, to taste

Preheat your slow cooker, following the manufacturer's instructions.

Put the vegetables and broth into the slow cooker and season well.

Set to Low and cook for 6 hours (or you can cook on High for 3–4 hours).

Twenty minutes before serving, add the crumbled cheese and stir well. Use a stick blender to blitz the soup until smooth.

Serve immediately.

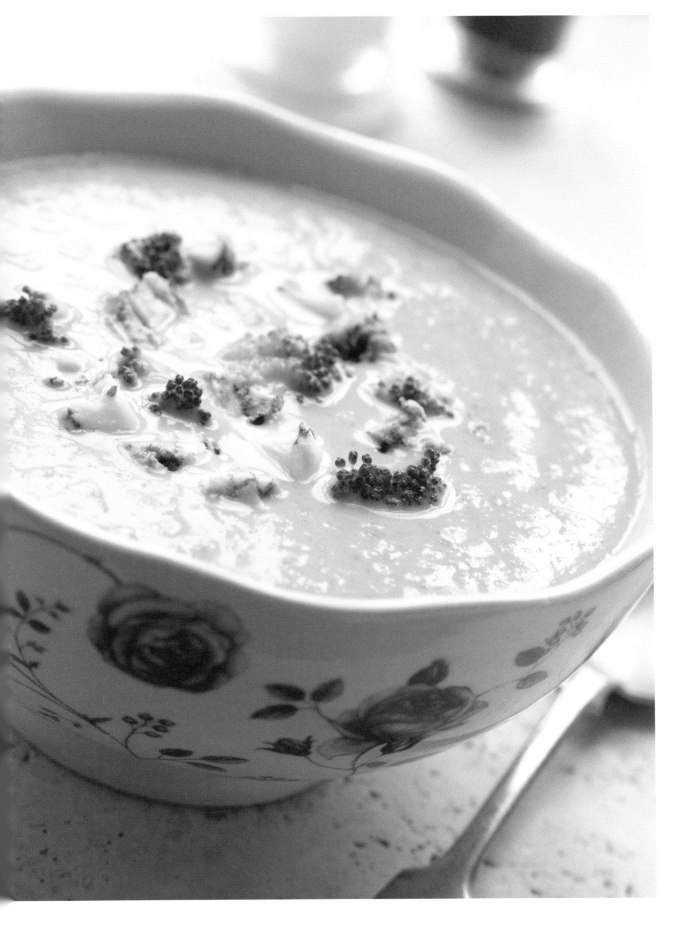

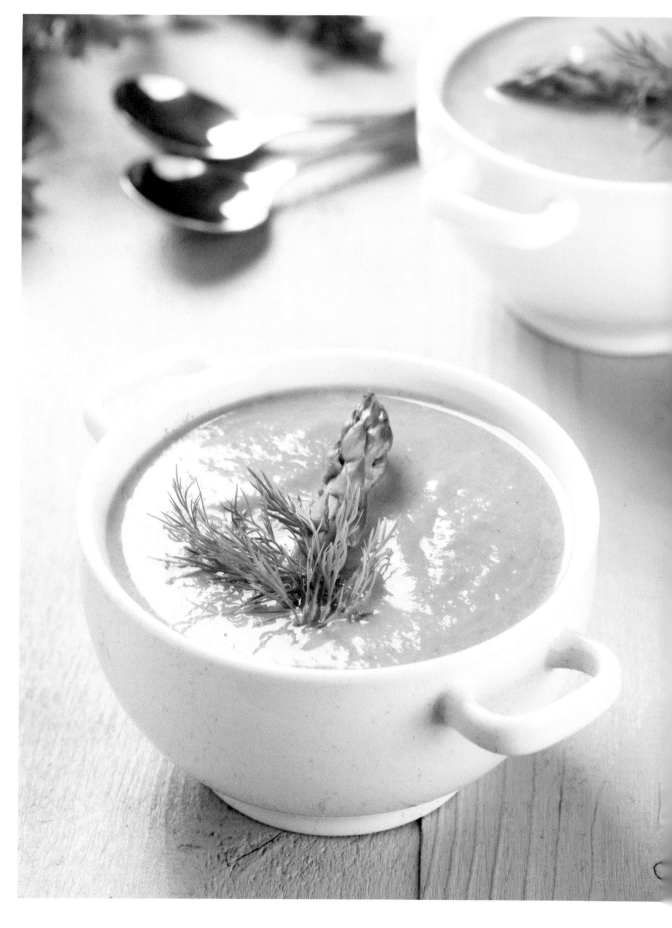

You can buy asparagus all year around, but it is at its tastiest, and most affordable, when in season. This is a lovely creamy soup which is surprisingly filling. It is delicious served with some crunchy bacon crumbled on the top.

Asparagus Soup

Serves 4

Nutritional information per serving
306 Kcals
26g fat
6.9g net carbohydrates
9.7g protein

Ingredients
500g asparagus, chopped

1 onion, finely chopped

450ml vegetable broth (or use bone or chicken broth if not vegetarian)

3 egg yolks

200ml crème fraîche (or use coconut cream if dairy-free)

black pepper, to taste

2 tbsp chopped fresh parsley

Preheat your slow cooker, following the manufacturer's instructions.

Put the asparagus and onion into your slow cooker. Add the broth and season well with black pepper

Set to High and cook for 2 hours.

Use a stick blender to whizz the soup (still in the slow cooker) until smooth.

Beat the egg yolks and crème fraîche together. Remove the lid of the slow cooker and very quickly add the crème fraiche mixture while stirring quickly to ensure the mix is dispersed but does not go lumpy.

Cook for another 15 minutes, then garnish with fresh parsley and serve.

I love the flavour of this soup. It is rich, creamy and very filling. If you are not a fan of very garlicky flavours, you can cut down on the number of cloves here.

Cauliflower, Garlic and Blue Cheese Soup

Serves 4

Nutritional information per serving
232 Kcals
16g fat
6.9g net carbohydrates
15g protein

Ingredients
4 garlic cloves, finely chopped

1 celery stick, finely chopped

1 large cauliflower, florets roughly chopped

600ml hot bone, chicken or vegetable broth

200g Danish blue cheese, plus extra to garnish

salt and black pepper, to taste

a small handful of chopped fresh parsley

Preheat your slow cooker or multi-cooker, following the manufacturer's instructions.

Put the garlic, celery and cauliflower into the slow cooker and pour over the hot broth.

Set to Low and cook for 6 hours.

Thirty minutes before serving, add the blue cheese and stir well until dissolved, then use a stick blender to whizz the soup until smooth.

Season to taste before serving. Garnish with the remaining crumbled blue cheese and chopped fresh parsley.

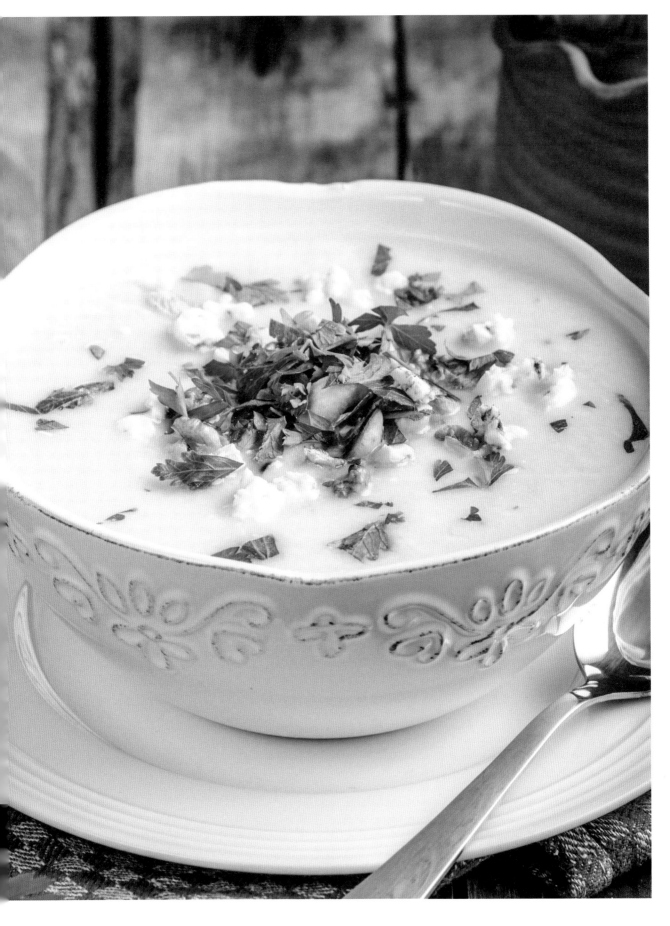

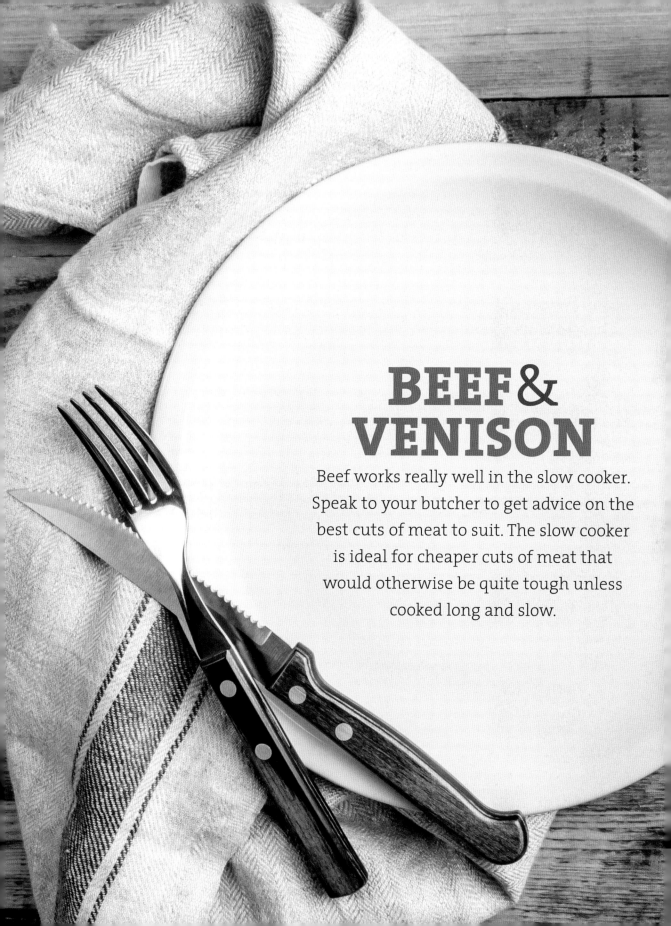

BEEF & VENISON

Beef works really well in the slow cooker. Speak to your butcher to get advice on the best cuts of meat to suit. The slow cooker is ideal for cheaper cuts of meat that would otherwise be quite tough unless cooked long and slow.

TOP TIPS

- Most of the recipes in this chapter ask for stewing steak, which is also known as braising steak (or chuck steak in the US). You can also use brisket, which is a tad more fatty, but is still an excellent choice for slow-cooking and a little more economical.
- Oxtail needs a long cook to make it tender but is bursting with flavour, which is often enhanced when eaten the day after cooking.
- I have included a handful of venison recipes in this chapter but it can be swapped for beef if you can't get hold of it. Venison is meat from deer; it's darker than beef with a great flavour. Most venison is not as gamey as it used to be as it is not subjected to the traditional maturing process that increases the flavour. The flavour also changes depending on what the animal eats – farmed, corn-fed deer have a less gamey taste than traditional wild deer. Venison is very nutrient-dense, but does not contain as much fat as beef and is high in protein.
- You will also notice that I have added liver or kidney to a few of these recipes. I know that some people don't like the thought of eating offal, but these foods are so nutrient-dense it would be foolish for me not to include them.
- Avoid using minced meat for long cooks, although it works well in the slow cooker for a reduced time.
- All the recipes in this chapter include the option of sautéing the beef prior to slow-cooking. This is not essential but it does help to seal the meat and enhance the flavour. Multi-cookers and some slow cookers have a sauté function but if yours does not, simply use a sauté pan on your hob and transfer to the slow cooker when browned.

My husband loves traditional food and steak and kidney pie is one of his favourites. I don't make a base for my pie, choosing instead to cook the steak and kidney filling in the slow cooker and then bake with the pastry top in the oven for 20–30 minutes. Top Tip: You can prepare the steak and kidney in the slow cooker the day before.

Keto Steak and Kidney Pie

Serves 4

Nutritional information per serving
443 Kcals
26g fat
4.7g net carbohydrates
45g protein

You will need
Baking parchment,
28–30cm pie dish

Ingredients
1 tbsp coconut or almond flour

2 tsp paprika

½ tsp mustard powder

500g stewing steak, diced

200g ox kidneys, diced

1 tbsp coconut oil

1 red onion, chopped

½ tsp dried marjoram

½ tsp dried thyme

350ml hot bone or beef broth, plus extra if needed

1 tbsp yeast extract

salt and black pepper, to taste

Preheat your slow cooker, following the manufacturer's instructions.

Put the coconut or almond flour, paprika and mustard powder in a bowl and mix to combine. Add the diced steak and kidneys and toss in the flour until it is well coated.

If your slow cooker has a sauté function, use this to heat the coconut oil; if not, use a sauté pan on your hob over a medium heat. Add the meat and fry gently in batches until it has browned all over. Return all the browned meat to the slow cooker along with the remaining ingredients and combine well.

Set to Low and cook for 6–7 hours. Add more broth if it starts to look dry.

You can prepare the pastry in advance and leave it in the fridge until ready to roll out and bake. To make the pastry put the butter, ground almonds and coconut flour into a food processor and whizz until it forms breadcrumbs. Add 1 of the eggs and whizz again, adding just enough cold water so that it forms a firm ball of dough. You may not need all the water, so just add a little at at time. Wrap the dough in clingfilm and leave in the fridge to chill until needed.

Preheat the oven to 180°C (160°C fan) Gas 4.

Roll out the pastry to a thickness of about 3mm. I find it easier to roll out between two sheets of baking parchment lightly dusted with coconut flour as keto pastry can be very delicate.

Place the steak and kidney into your deep pie dish. Beat the remaining egg and brush a little around the edge of the dish to help the pastry stick. Top with the pastry, pressing down on to the edge of the pastry dish and trim. Brush with the remaining egg to glaze.

Bake the pie in the oven for 20–30 minutes until the pastry is golden and crisp.

Serve with steamed green vegetables.

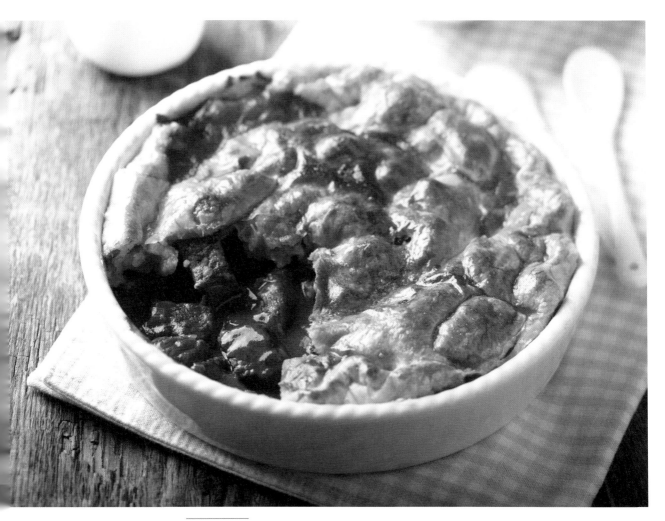

For the keto pastry

30g butter (or use coconut oil if dairy-free)

120g ground almonds

40g coconut flour

2 eggs

4–6 tbsp cold water

Top Tip
You can prepare the steak and kidney in the slow cooker the day before.

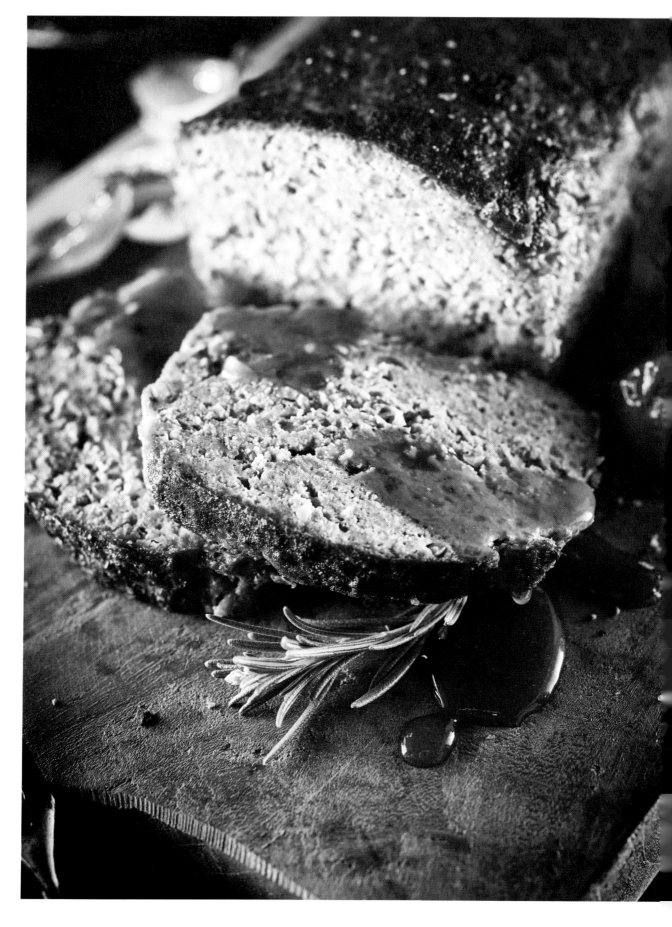

This is a popular meal in the US, but it's so tasty we ought to adopt it more in the UK. It works brilliantly in the slow cooker and also freezes well, so why not double up the recipe? I serve this with a delicious green salad in the warmer months and with comforting steamed vegetables and a cauliflower mash in the winter months. This is very filling so you don't need very thick slices!

Beef and Bacon Meatloaf

Serves 6

Nutritional information per serving
435 Kcals
30g fat
6g net carbohydrates
33g protein

Ingredients
750g beef mince

150g back bacon, lardons or pancetta, finely chopped

50g ground almonds

1 onion, finely chopped

2 garlic cloves, crushed

2 tsp dried oregano

1 tsp paprika

1 tsp dried thyme

1 tbsp yeast extract

salt and black pepper, to taste

1 egg, beaten

2 tbsp tomato purée (optional)

1 tbsp coconut aminos (optional)

Preheat your slow cooker, following the manufacturer's instructions.

Put the beef mince into a large bowl, add all the ingredients (except the tomato purée and coconut aminos) and combine well.

Use your hands to shape the mixture into a loaf. Place a rack in the base of the slow cooker – if you don't have a rack, roll up some foil into long sausage shapes and place these on the base – this helps the fat drain away from the loaf. (If you are worried about lifting out the loaf, fold a long piece of foil lengthways and place this under the loaf before you place the loaf on the rack [or foil base], leaving enough either side to lift the loaf out when cooked.)

Set the slow cooker to Low and cook for 5–6 hours.

Carefully remove the loaf from the slow cooker – it can be quite fragile so handle with care.

If you want to brown the top of the loaf, mix the tomato purée with the coconut aminos and brush over the loaf. Place under a preheated grill for 10 minutes until golden.

Serve hot or cold, cut into slices.

Top Tip
I have used beef in this recipe but you can use pork or a combination of the two.

For those who have never had this dish, it is just like a beef version of lamb shanks where the meat just melts off the bone. The sauce is made with a little red wine to add depth and flavour, however if you prefer not to use wine, you can just add more of the bone/beef broth. This wholesome dish really does need to be served with a celeriac or cauliflower mash and steamed vegetables or, for a dinner party treat, try my dauphinoise celeriac (see page 147).

Braised Short Beef Ribs

Serves 4

Nutritional information per serving
556 Kcals
31g fat
5.6g net carbohydrates
46g protein

Ingredients
4–8 beef short ribs (depending on size)

1 onion, diced

2 garlic cloves, roughly chopped

1 celery stick, diced

1 tbsp tomato purée

250g smoked pancetta, cubed

375ml burgundy red wine or bone or beef broth

1 tsp dried thyme

½ tsp dried rosemary

1 heaped tsp paprika

3 dried bay leaves

Preheat your slow cooker, following the manufacturer's instructions.

Some people like to brown the ribs before they pop them into the slow cooker. I really don't think this is necessary, but if you prefer to do this, do it now, either by using the sauté function on your slow cooker or by using a sauté pan on your hob.

Place the ribs into the slow cooker and add all the remaining ingredients.

Set to Low and cook for 8 hours.

When you are ready to serve, you can thicken the liquid if necessary, by removing the ribs and bay leaves and pouring the broth into a pan (or switch to sauté function if you have a multi-cooker). Heat until it starts to thicken and reduce.

Serve with celeriac or cauliflower mash and steamed vegetables, with the reduced sauce poured over the ribs.

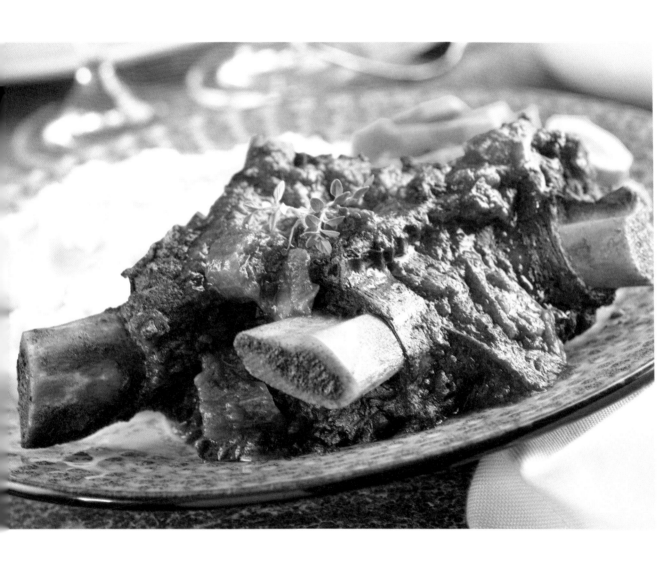

Oxtail is an inexpensive but really flavoursome cut that is packed with nutrients, especially iron. This recipe is ideal for a dinner party served with celeriac mash and steamed green vegetables. Get your butcher to prepare the oxtail and cut into pieces for you.

Oxtail and Bacon Casserole

Serves 6
❄ ⊘

Nutritional information per serving
576 Kcals
34g fat
8.9g net carbohydrates
47g protein

Ingredients
1 tbsp coconut or almond flour

1 tbsp paprika

1kg oxtail, cut into pieces

1–2 tsp olive oil or coconut oil

350g cooking bacon or lardons, thickly diced

3 garlic cloves, crushed

1 celery stick, diced

8 radishes, halved

1 small carrot, diced

400ml bone or beef broth

175ml port

2 tbsp tomato purée

2 tsp dried thyme

2 bay leaves

salt and pepper, to taste

Preheat your slow cooker, following the manufacturer's instructions.

Put the coconut or almond flour and paprika into a bowl and combine well. Dip the oxtail pieces into the flour until lightly coated.

If your slow cooker has a sauté function, you can use this; if not, use a sauté pan on your hob. Heat the olive or coconut oil, add the oxtail and bacon and cook until the meat is brown, sealing in the flavour. Transfer to the slow cooker, along with any juices.

Add all the remaining ingredients and season to taste.

Set to Low and cook for 8 hours.

Remove the bay leaves before serving with celeriac mash and green steamed vegetables.

This stew combines two flavoursome and nourishing meats. Venison has a wonderful rich flavour and works brilliantly in the slow cooker. Liver is packed with nutrients – it really should be classed as a superfood. It provides high levels of B vitamins – it is a particularly rich sources of B12 – along with vitmain A, iron, copper and choline. Not only does it have great nutritional credentials, it also tastes great when slow cooked.

Venison, Juniper and Liver Stew

Serves 4
❄ ⊘

Nutritional information per serving
293 Kcals
6.8g fat
7.1g net carbohydrates
49g protein

Ingredients
500g venison, cut into large chunks

400g calves livers, diced

2 garlic cloves, chopped

1 red onion, diced

1 tbsp tomato purée

1 tbsp juniper berries, crushed

1 tsp dried thyme

½ tsp dried rosemary

1 tsp dried parsley

1 bay leaf

500ml bone or beef broth, plus extra as needed

salt and black pepper, to taste

Preheat your slow cooker, following the manufacturer's recommendations.

You can seal the meat by frying it in a sauté pan with a little coconut oil, although this isn't strictly necessary. However, if your slow cooker has a sauté function or you have a multi-cooker, you can do this without having to use another pan.

Add all the remaining ingredients to the slow cooker and combine well.

Set to Low and cook for 6–8 hours until the venison and liver is very tender. Add more broth if it starts to look dry.

Serve with cauliflower mash and steamed green vegetables.

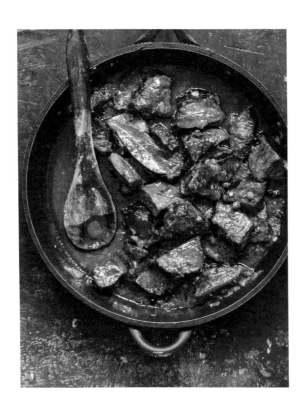

This is my take on Italian meatballs. I love food with a little kick and preparing an arrabbiata sauce to accompany these meatballs makes them extremely tasty. Traditionally you would use dried chillies for an arrabbiata sauce, but I use fresh in my recipe. If you like heat, you could also add some fresh chillies to the meatball mixture.

Arrabbiata Meatballs

Serves 4

Nutritional information per serving
406 Kcals
27g fat
7g net carbohydrates
32g protein

For the sauce
400g tin chopped tomatoes

1 red onion, finely chopped

3 garlic cloves, crushed

2 red chillies (to taste), finely chopped

4 tsp dried oregano

1 tsp dried basil

1 tsp dried thyme

salt and black pepper, to taste

For the meatballs
500g beef mince

1 egg

1 tsp paprika

40g grated Parmesan (optional; omit if dairy-free)

2 tsp olive or coconut oil

Preheat your slow cooker, following the manufacturer's instructions.

Put all the sauce ingredients into the slow cooker and stir until combined. Set to High while you prepare the meatballs.

Put the mince into a bowl. Add the egg and the paprika and season to taste. Add the Parmesan (if using) and mix everything together with your hands until combined.

Using damp hands (to stop the mixture sticking), roll the mixture into your meatballs – you should get 12–16 meatballs, depending on size.

Heat a little olive or coconut oil in a sauté pan on the hob and fry the meatballs – just to seal them, not to cook them right through.

Once sealed, transfer to the slow cooker. Turn down to Low and cook for 5 hours.

Serve on a bed of courgette spaghetti.

Top Tip
This is a great recipe to double up and freeze. Put the uncooked meatballs on a baking sheet and place in the freezer until frozen, then bag them up in a ziplock bag. Defrost thoroughly before using.

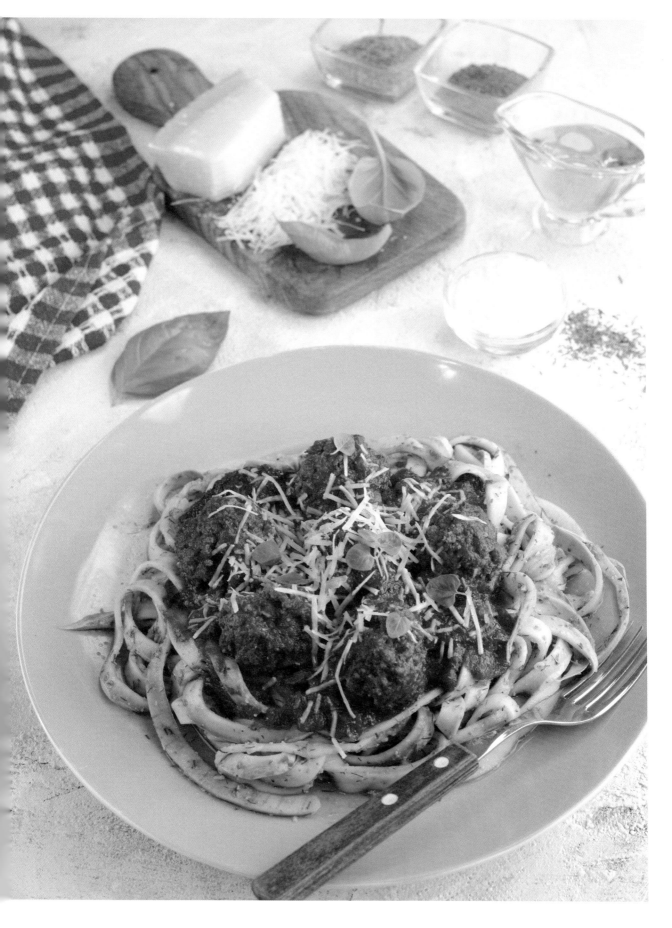

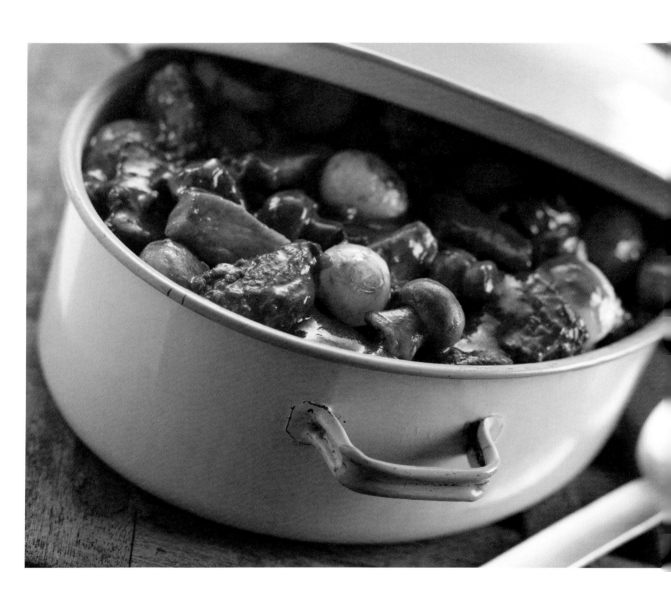

I always used beef to make my bourguignon but was given some venison and decided to try it instead for one of my family's favourite recipes. It worked brilliantly, adding an extra depth of flavour. It can be made in advance, even a day or two before required, as it does improve with age. I serve this with celeriac dauphinoise and steamed green vegetables.

Rich Venison Bourguignon

Serves 6
❄ ⊘

Nutritional information per serving
509 Kcals
26g fat
4.8g net carbohydrates
52g protein

Ingredients
750g beef braising steak, diced

1–2 tbsp coconut flour

1 tsp olive or coconut oil

1 onion, diced

2 garlic cloves, roughly chopped

250g thick smoked pancetta, diced

400g tin chopped tomatoes

400ml burgundy red wine

1 tsp dried thyme

½ tsp dried rosemary

2 heaped tsp paprika

150g button mushrooms, halved

1–3 tsp coconut flour, arrowroot or xanthan gum (optional, to thicken)

Preheat your slow cooker, following your manfacturer's instructions.

Toss the beef in the coconut flour until lightly coated all over.

Heat the olive or coconut oil and sear the beef until browned. If your slow cooker has a sauté function, use this; if not, use a sauté pan over a medium heat on your hob.

Transfer the beef to the slow cooker and add all the remaining ingredients except the mushrooms; combine well.

Set to Low and cook for 8 hours.

Half an hour before you are ready to serve, add the mushrooms, stirring well so they are submerged. Turn to High and cook for 30 minutes. If you need to thicken the sauce, mix 1–3 tsp coconut flour, arrowroot or xanthan gum with water and add this to the slow cooker when you add the mushrooms.

Serve with my delicious baked celeriac dauphinoise (see page 147) and steamed green leafy vegetables.

A traditional dish, given a keto twist. This is comfort on a plate. I always make more as it is delicious for a lunch the following day. You don't have to do the fancy cauliflower or celeriac mash piping on the top, you can just smooth all the mash over the mince. I always remove from the slow cooker and pop under the grill with a sprinkle of cheese to brown.

Cottage Pie

Serves 6

Nutritional values
436 kcals
30g fat
7.4g of net carbohydrates
33g protein

Ingredients
1 tsp coconut oil

1 red onion, chopped

2 garlic cloves, finely chopped

750g beef mince

75g mushrooms, diced

2–3 tsp yeast extract

1 tbsp tomato purée

300ml hot beef bone broth

2 tsp dried thyme

1 tsp dried marjoram

1 tsp paprika

salt and black pepper, to taste

For the mash
1 large head of cauliflower (or celeriac if you prefer)

25g butter

100g mature Cheddar, grated

Preheat your slow cooker, following the manufacturer's instructions.

If you have a sauté function, use that to heat the coconut oil and sauté the onion for 1–2 minutes; if not, use a sauté pan on your hob.

Add the garlic and mince and cook for 5 minutes.

Switch to slow cooker mode and set to High (or transfer to the slow cooker if you were using a hob). Add all remaining ingredients and combine well. Leave to cook on High while you prepare the mash.

Cook the cauliflower in a steamer until soft and then mash. Stir in the butter and the Cheddar – if you like a cheesy topping, keep some of the cheese back. Season to taste.

Pipe or spoon the mash over the top of the mince: either press the mash down and finish with a pattern made using your fork, or spoon two-thirds of the mash on to the top of pie and smooth over before piping over the remaining third. Cook on High for 2 hours or on Low for 4–5 hours.

When you are ready to serve, top with the remaining grated cheese and place under a hot grill until golden.

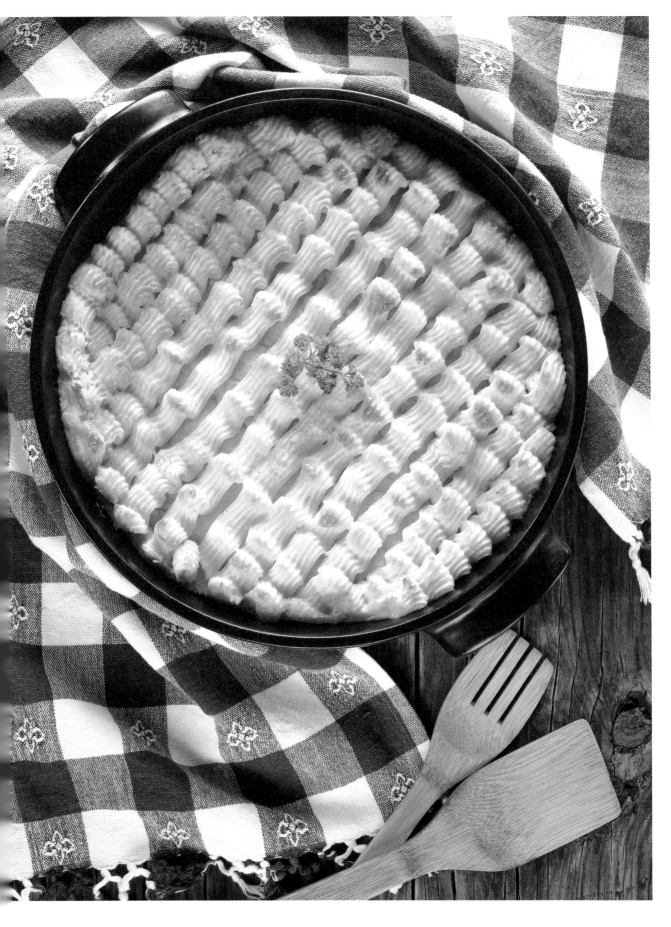

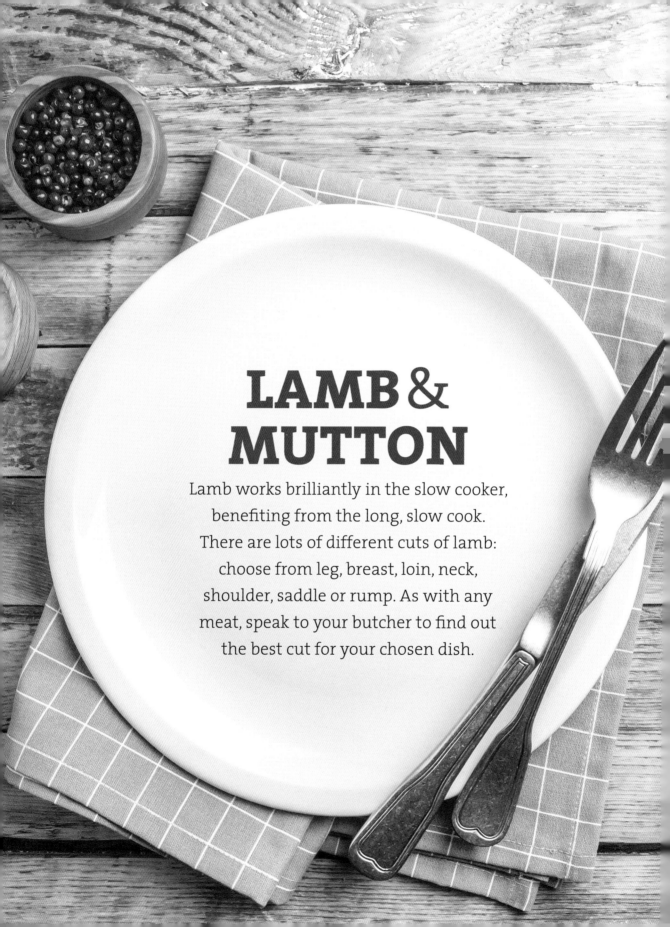

LAMB & MUTTON

Lamb works brilliantly in the slow cooker, benefiting from the long, slow cook. There are lots of different cuts of lamb: choose from leg, breast, loin, neck, shoulder, saddle or rump. As with any meat, speak to your butcher to find out the best cut for your chosen dish.

The term lamb only applies to a young lamb. Although lamb is readily available all year around, we often hear about spring lamb – this is a tender meat but does lack the flavour of autumn lamb. After about 2 years old a lamb is then known as mutton; it has a stronger flavour, almost gamey in taste, and works well for slow cooking. I have used the name lamb in these recipes, but you can also use mutton – it works particularly well in curries.

You will find recipes such as lamb shanks, lamb chops and hotpot in this chapter (lamb shanks is one of my favourites and is delicious when slow-cooked). Diced lamb is used for most of the casserole, ragout, curry or tagine dishes.

I use lamb in this recipe but it works just as well with beef (or even chicken). Remember, you can use mutton instead of lamb for a deeper flavour and this works brilliantly with curries. This is a quick and easy recipe as long as you have a food processor to help make the curry paste.

Lamb Rendang Curry

Serves 6
❄ Ⓘ

Nutritional information per serving
420 Kcals
30g fat
6.6g net carbohydrates
30g protein

Ingredients
2 tsp coconut oil

750g diced lamb (such as boneless shoulder) or mutton, cut into large chunks

1 large red onion, roughly chopped

coriander leaves, to garnish

For the curry paste
4cm piece of fresh ginger

4 garlic cloves

3 chillies, or to taste

2 lemongrass stalks, hard outer leaves removed

4cm piece of fresh galangal

4 cardamom pods

4 kaffir lime leaves

1 tsp fennel seeds

2 tsp coriander seeds

1 tsp cumin seeds

grated zest and juice of 1 lime

2 tsp ground cinnamon

½ tsp ground ginger

1 tsp hot paprika

1 tsp ground turmeric

400ml tin full-fat coconut milk

Put all the curry paste ingredients into your food processor and whizz until well combined and you have a smooth paste.

Preheat your slow cooker, following the manufacturer's instructions.

If your slow cooker has a sauté function, you can use this; if not, use a sauté pan on your hob. Heat the coconut oil, add the lamb pieces and cook until brown, sealing in the flavour. Transfer to the slow cooker.

Add the curry paste and chopped red onion. Combine well, set to Low and cook for 8 hours. Add more liquid (coconut milk, water, or broth) if needed.

Garnish with fresh coriander and serve with cauliflower or broccoli rice and keto flatbreads.

Top Tip
Double up the curry paste and store in the freezer ready to pop out whenever you fancy a curry.

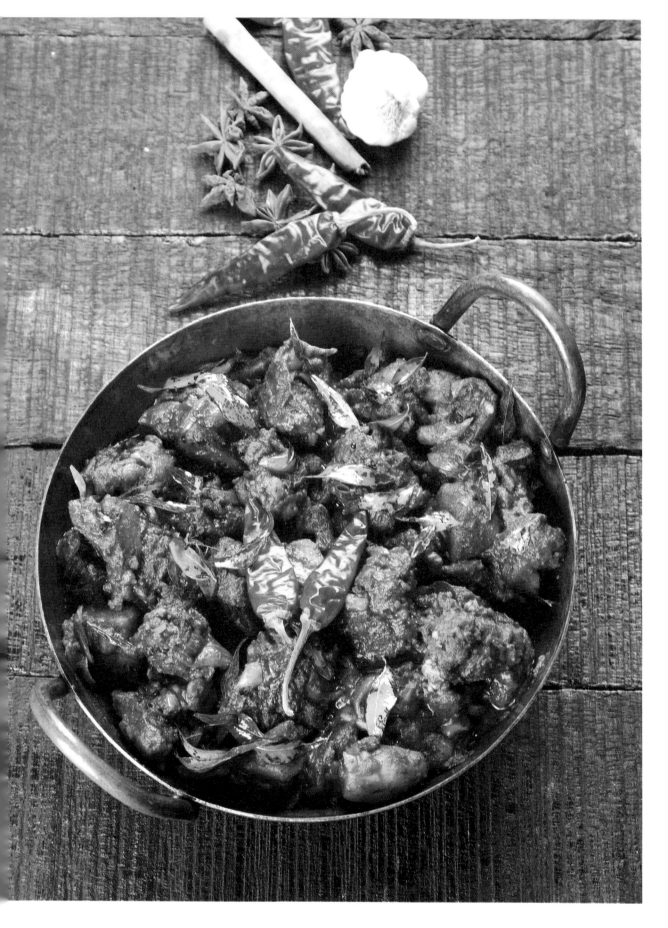

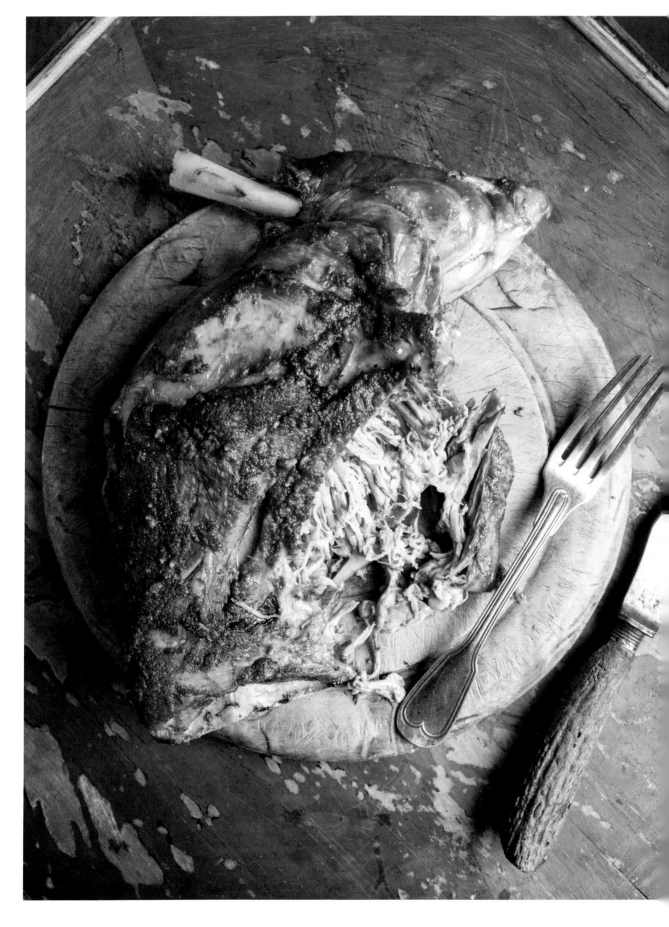

This is really a tasty lamb version of pulled pork. The shredded lamb is great with steamed vegetables and mash or served with a lovely salad. It is also great in my keto wraps (see page 156) for a tasty packed lunch treat.

Shredded Lamb

Serves 4–6

Nutritional information per serving (based on serving 4)
130 Kcals
9.4g fat
6.8g net carbohydrates
4g protein

Ingredients
1.5kg lamb leg or shoulder

2 garlic cloves

1 red chilli

2 tsp dried rosemary

1 tsp dried thyme

1 tsp dried mint

1 tbsp Dijon mustard

2 tbsp olive oil

2 red onions, sliced

400ml hot bone, lamb or chicken broth

salt and black pepper, to taste

Preheat your slow cooker, following the manufacturer's recommendations.

Use a sharp knife to make incisions all over the lamb leg or shoulder.

Put the garlic, chilli, herbs and mustard into a food processor. Add the olive oil and pulse for 30 seconds.

Rub this mixture over the lamb shoulder, making sure it soaks into the cut slits. If you like a more potent garlic flavour, slice a couple more garlic cloves and push these into the incisions. Season well to taste.

Place the onion slices into the base of the slow cooker. Pour in the broth before carefully adding the lamb shoulder so its sits on the bed of onions and broth.

Set to Low and cook for 8–10 hours.

Remove from the slow cooker and carefully shred the meat to use as required.

Traditionally a lamb hotpot contains lots of root vegetables and is topped with a layer of potato. It is absolutely delicious so naturally I got thinking about how to tweak it to make it suitable for the ketogenic diet. Celeriac is a great substitute for potato so that solves the top – it has a lovely taste similar to parsnip. The recipe uses bone broth, but if you want to boost the flavour do add a sugar-free lamb stock gel or cube.

Keto Lamb Hotpot

Serves 6

❄ ⊘

Nutritional information per serving
364 Kcals
19g fat
6.8g net carbohydrates
39g protein

Ingredients
2 tbsp coconut flour

1 tsp paprika

750g stewing lamb, diced

2 lamb kidneys (about 250g), diced

1 tbsp coconut oil or butter

2 onions, finely chopped

1 carrot, diced

½ celeriac, thinly sliced

450ml hot bone broth

2 tsp dried thyme

2 tsp dried rosemary

2 tsp dried mint

salt and black pepper, to taste

a handful of grated Cheddar (optional)

Preheat your slow cooker, following the manufacturer's instructions.

Put the flour and paprika into a large bowl and combine well. Add the lamb and kidneys and toss to coat in the flour, then put to one side.

If your slow cooker has a sauté option, you can use this, if not, use a sauté pan on your hob. Heat the coconut oil or butter, add the meat and cook until browned, sealing in the flavour. Transfer to the slow cooker.

Add the onions and carrot and mix together, then top with the sliced celeriac.

Mix the broth with the herbs and some salt and pepper and pour this over the vegetables and celeriac slices.

Set to Low and cook for 7–8 hours.

If you want to brown off the celeriac, you can place it under a grill. For added flavour, sprinkle with some grated cheese before grilling (if you are not dairy-free).

Serve with shredded steamed cabbage.

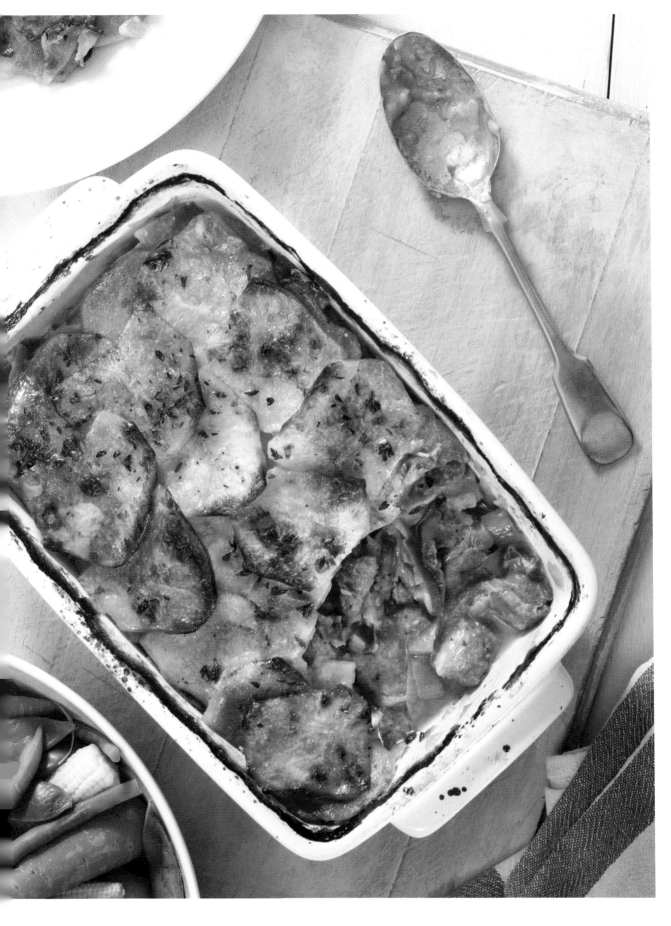

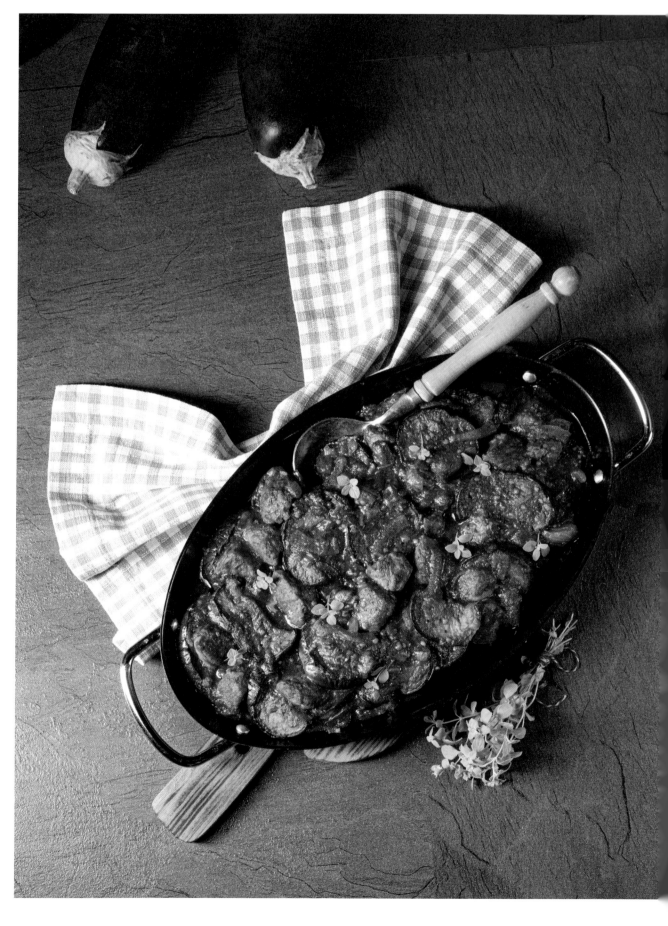

This is my version of the Greek dish *arni me melitzanes*, which I believe means lamb and aubergine casserole. This is a really tasty dish, with garlic, olives, peppers and aubergine as a fabulous accompaniment to the lamb. I serve this with cauliflower rice and finish with crumbled feta or goat's cheese. This recipe also goes well served with my cheesy garlic bread (see page 159).

Mediterranean Lamb

Serves 4

Nutritional information per serving
454 Kcals
27g fat
9.5g net carbohydrates
31g protein

Ingredients
500g stewing lamb, diced

1 small red onion, finely chopped

2 garlic cloves, crushed

1 red pepper, finely diced

2 aubergines, sliced

400g tin chopped tomatoes

75g pitted black olives, quartered

3 tsp dried oregano

½ tsp dried basil

½ tsp dried rosemary

2 tbsp sun-dried tomato paste

200ml red wine or bone broth

salt and black pepper, to taste

Preheat your slow cooker, following the manufacturer's instructions.

Put all the ingredients into the slow cooker and set to Low. Cook for 8 hours until the lamb is cooked and tender. Season to taste.

Serve with cauliflower rice and a green salad. For a lovely touch, finish with a sprinkle of crumbled feta or goat's cheese (if you are not dairy-free).

I know lamb shanks are traditionally cooked in a lovely, rich wine sauce, but I fancied a change one day – I also wanted to use up some of my curry paste – so I decided to mix the two together. These shanks are tender and packed with flavour.

Indian Spiced Lamb Shanks

Serves 4–6

ⓧ

Nutritional information per serving (based on serving 4)
690 Kcals
44g fat
9.7g net carbohydrates
62g protein

Ingredients
1 tsp coconut oil (optional)

4 lamb shanks (about 1.2kg in total)

1 red onion, finely chopped

4 tbsp everyday curry paste (see page 174)

400g tin chopped tomatoes

grated zest and juice of 1 lime

300ml hot bone or lamb broth

a small handful of fresh coriander

2–3 tbsp coconut cream (optional)

Preheat your slow cooker, following the manufacturer's instructions.

If your slow cooker has a sauté function use it to brown off the lamb shanks in the coconut oil; if not, use a sauté pan set over a medium heat on your hob. When they are browned on all sides, after 2–3 minutes, transfer to your slow cooker. I don't always bother with this step as my family often don't notice any difference!

Add all the remaining ingredients to the slow cooker, except for the coconut cream and coriander.

Set to Low and cook for 8–10 hours until the lamb is cooked and starting to come away from the bone. Thirty minutes before you are ready to serve add the chopped coriander.

Remove the lamb shanks from the slow cooker and put to one side, covered in foil to keep warm. Strain the sauce through a sieve into a saucepan and heat until it starts to reduce and thicken. If you like a creamier sauce, add a few tablespoons of coconut cream and stir until warmed through.

Serve the lamb shanks topped with some of the sauce and finish with a scattering of coriander leaves. Enjoy with some cauliflower rice and keto flatbreads (see page 159).

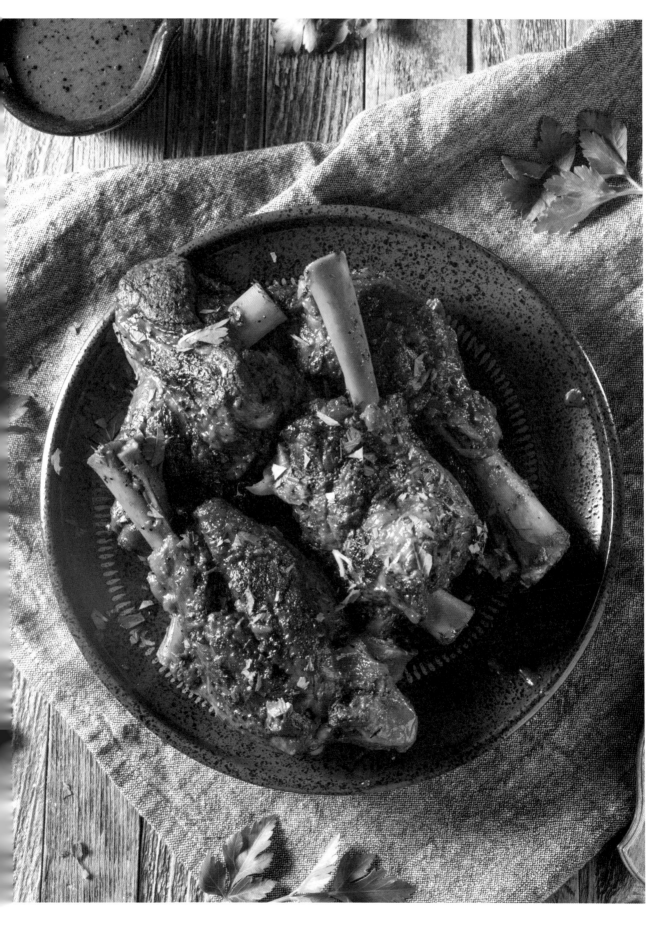

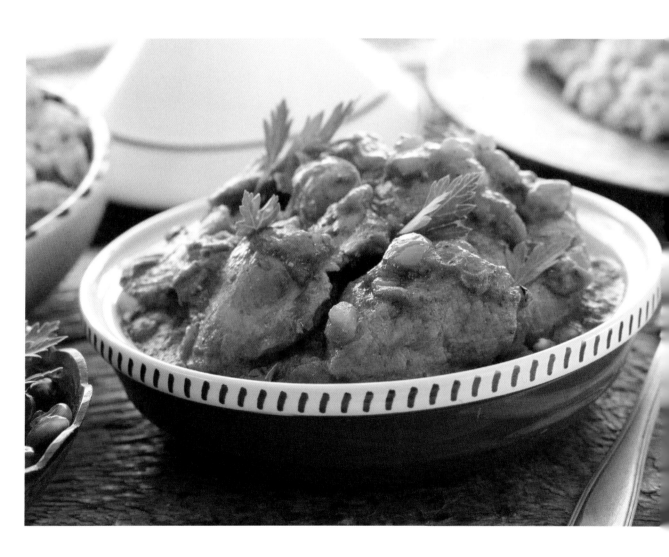

Traditionally this recipe would include chickpeas and dried apricots but as this is a keto version, you do need a little artistic licence. This recipe works well with mutton instead of lamb for a deeper flavour. I use my harissa paste in this recipe (see page 169). This is wonderful served with cauliflower rice.

Moroccan Lamb

Serves 6

Nutritional information per serving
339 Kcals
20g fat
7g net carbohydrates
31g protein

Ingredients
1 tsp coconut oil

750g stewing lamb or mutton, cut into chunks

1 onion, diced

1 red or yellow pepper

2–3cm piece of fresh ginger, roughly chopped

2 garlic cloves, roughly chopped

4 tbsp Spiced Harissa Paste (see page 169)

1 tsp ground cinnamon

½ tsp ground ginger

400g tin chopped tomatoes

300ml hot bone, lamb or vegetable broth

salt and black pepper, to taste

fresh coriander leaves, to garnish

Preheat your slow cooker, following the manufacturer's instructions.

If your slow cooker has a sauté function, use it to heat the coconut oil and brown the lamb pieces; if not use a sauté pan over a medium heat on the hob. Transfer the browned lamb to the slow cooker.

Add all the remaining ingredients.

Set to Low and cook for 8–10 hours.

Finish with a sprinkle of fresh coriander leaves. You can add some red jewel-like colour by adding some pomegranate seeds when serving.

Serve with cauliflower rice.

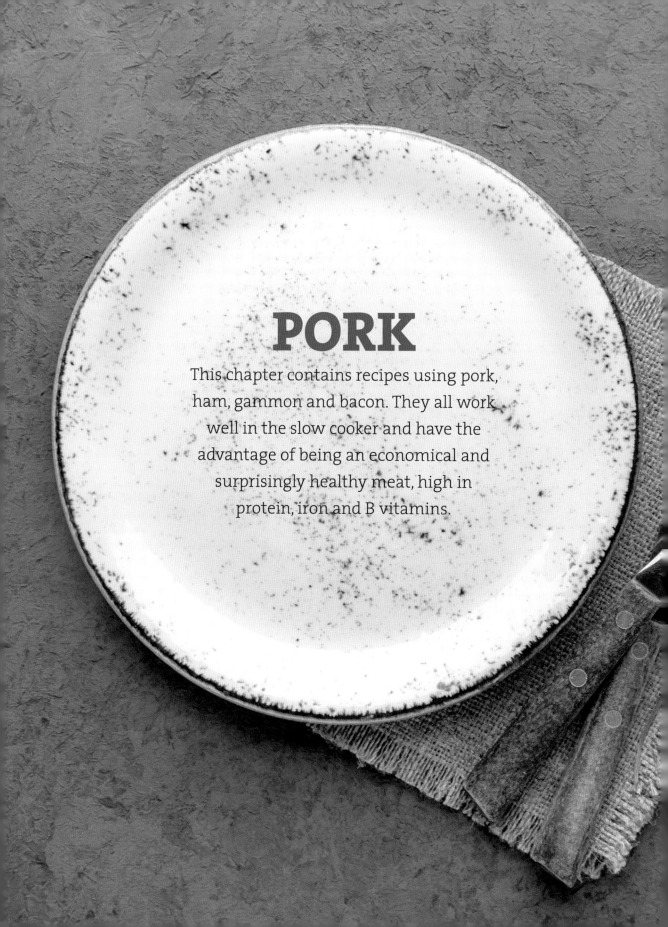

PORK

This chapter contains recipes using pork, ham, gammon and bacon. They all work well in the slow cooker and have the advantage of being an economical and surprisingly healthy meat, high in protein, iron and B vitamins.

Pork is cheap and you can buy lots of different cuts that work well in the slow cooker. I use pork belly, pork tenderloins, cheek and pork shoulder. Hocks are really affordable, tasty and work well in the slow cooker. Cook them in a similar way to how you would cook a ham or gammon joint. Speak to your butcher for cost-cutting suggestions that work well when slow-cooked.

GAMMON

I cook a gammon joint every week for my family. I have not included a recipe for this here as I have done this in other books; however, here are some basic instructions: simply place the gammon joint in the slow cooker, cover with water, set to Low and cook for 3–5 hours (timings depend on the size of the joint). If you want to crisp up the fat preheat the oven to 210°C (190°C fan) Gas 7 and roast the joint for 20–30 minutes after cooking. I use gammon for lunches and snacks during the week – one of my go-to lunches is scrambled eggs with slices of gammon.

These sticky, sweet barbecue ribs are delicious and literally melt off the bone. Please note, they are higher in carbs due to the sweeter sauce base. However, you can remove the ribs from the sauce after cooking which will lower the overall carb count. You can grill or barbecue these after slow-cooking to create a lovely crisp, charred effect on the ribs.

Barbecue Ribs

Serves 4

Nutritional information per serving
415 Kcals
25g fat
17g net carbohydrates
34g protein

Ingredients
2 tsp olive or coconut oil

700g ribs or thickly sliced pork loin

For the barbecue sauce
2 tbsp tomato purée

2 tbsp apple cider vinegar

70g Sukrin Gold granules or Sukrin Fibre Syrup (erythritol)

2 tsp smoked paprika

2 tsp Chinese five-spice

1 tsp liquid smoke (optional)

2cm piece of fresh ginger, grated

2 garlic cloves, crushed

grated zest of 1 lime

200ml water

salt and black pepper, to taste

Preheat your slow cooker, following the manufacturer's instructions.

If your slow cooker has a sauté function, you can use this; if not, use a sauté pan on your hob. Heat the olive or coconut oil, add the pork and cook until brown, sealing in the flavour (you can skip this step if you prefer). Transfer to the slow cooker.

Put all the barbecue sauce ingredients into a bowl and mix well until combined. Pour this over the pork .

Set to Low and cook for 6–7 hours.

Remove the pork from the slow cooker. If you want to serve with the sauce, transfer the liquid from the slow cooker to a saucepan and place over a medium heat until it has thickened to a syrupy sauce.

Place the pork on a serving plate with the sauce in a jug ready to add if needed.

Top Tip
Use the barbecue sauce ingredients as a marinade for your favourite meat; simply adjust the water content to form the consistency you desire. It will keep well in the fridge in a jar for up to 2 weeks.

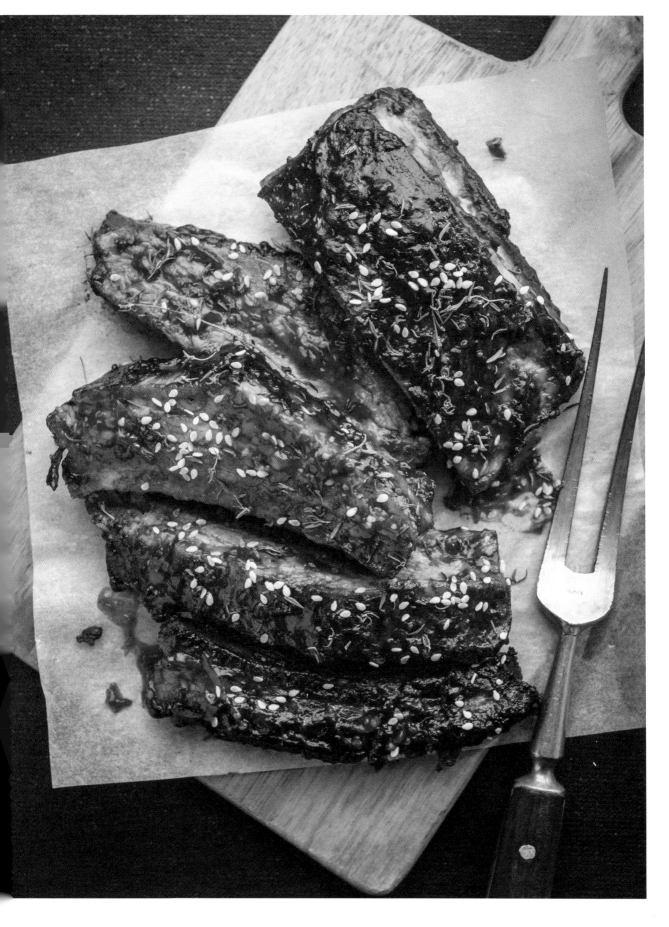

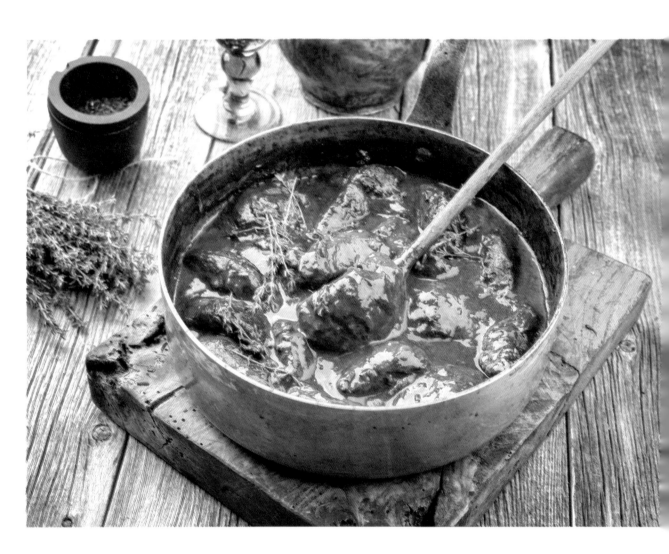

This is a lovely, rich, smoky casserole – pig cheeks are delicious after a long, slow cook. You can get these from your butcher and you can also swap them for beef or ox cheeks. This is delicious served with steamed savoy cabbage, cauliflower mash and a drizzle of soured cream.

Braised Pig Cheeks

Serves 6
❄ ⊘

Nutritional information per serving
398 Kcals
27g fat
7.5g net carbohydrates
29g protein

Ingredients
700g pig cheeks, halved if large

200g diced chorizo (or use lardons)

1 red onion, diced

2 garlic cloves, crushed

1–2 chillies, deseeded and finely chopped

1 red pepper, deseeded and diced

2 tsp smoked paprika

1 tsp dried parsley

1 tsp dried thyme

½ tsp dried marjoram

400g tin chopped tomatoes

1 tbsp tomato purée

200ml hot bone or chicken broth

salt and black pepper, to taste

Preheat your slow cooker, following the manufacturer's instructions.

Put all the ingredients into the slow cooker and combine well, seasoning to taste.

Set to Low and cook for 7–8 hours.

Taste and adjust the seasoning. Pig cheeks shred well once they have been slow-cooked, so if you prefer a casserole with shredded meat remove from the slow cooker, shred with two forks and then return the meat to the cooker.

Serve with steamed green vegetables.

This really is melt-in-the-mouth. I love the flavours of garlic, thyme and rosemary, with a touch of mustard in the gravy. This makes a wonderful change from a roast dinner; serve with roasted celeriac, creamy cauliflower cheese and some steamed vegetables. If you have any leftover pork, you can use this in the week as a curry.

Melt-in-the-mouth Pork Tenderloin

Serves 8

Nutritional information per serving
482 Kcals
36g fat
1.7g net carbohydrates
38g protein

Ingredients
1 large onion, sliced

1.5kg boneless pork loin joint

1 tsp coconut or olive oil

2 tsp dried thyme

2 tsp dried rosemary

2 tsp Dijon mustard

3 garlic cloves, chopped

350ml hot bone, pork or chicken broth

1 tsp xanthan gum (optional)

salt and black pepper, to taste

Preheat your slow cooker, following the manufacturer's instructions.

Arrange the sliced onion over the base of the slow cooker and add the pork loin so it is sitting on a bed of onions.

Mix the oil, thyme, rosemary, mustard and garlic together and spread this over the loin. Season well.

Carefully pour the broth to the side of the pork loin so as not to dislodge the herb mixture.

Set the slow cooker to Low and cook for 6 hours.

Remove the loin from the slow cooker and wrap in foil to rest. You can then use the liquid as a gravy if you wish. If you want to thicken it, transfer to a saucepan and heat gently until it starts to thicken and reduce. (You can also add a teaspoon of xanthan gum to thicken it, see my guide on thickening agents on page 189).

Serve with roasted celeriac and steamed vegetables.

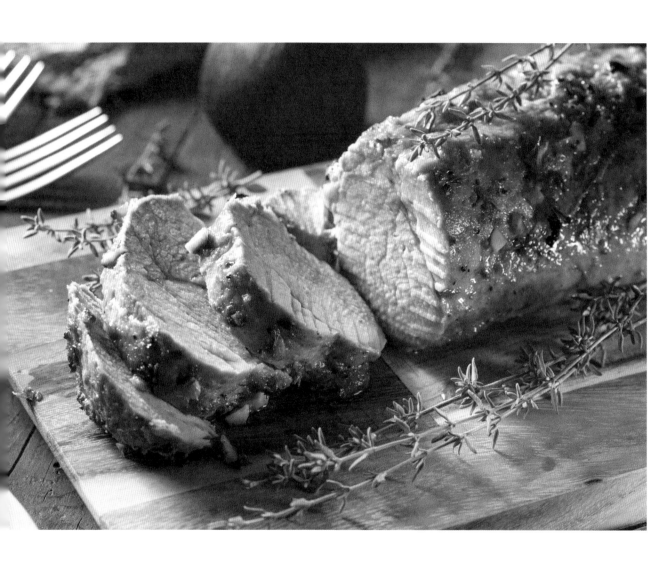

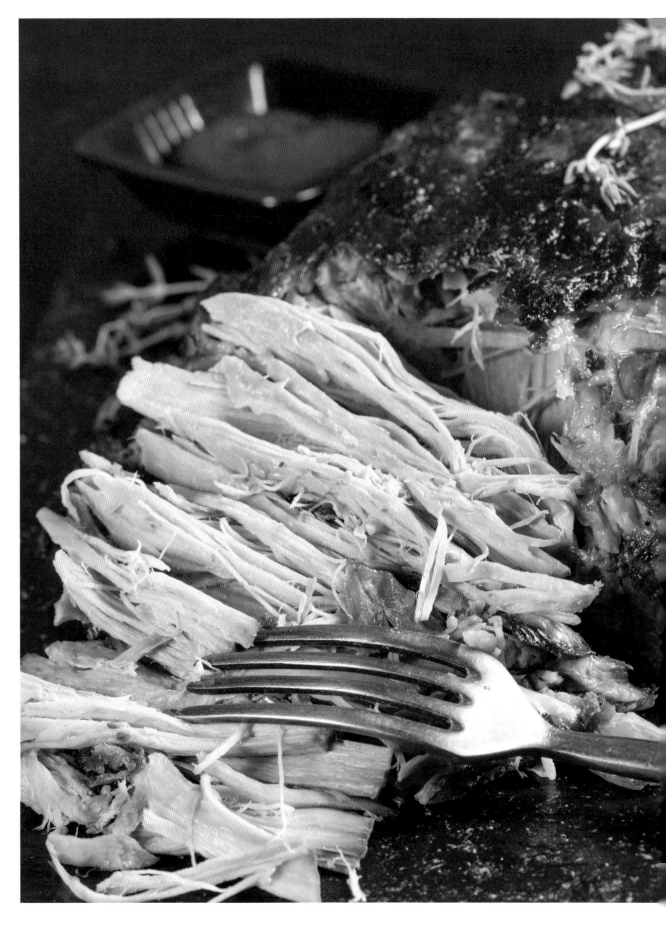

Pulled pork is a real classic and suits the slow cooker perfectly. Traditionally made with a sweet sauce, this is a keto version. I love this with salads, but you can, of course, go down a more conventional route and add your pulled pork to a keto bun or flaxseed wrap.

Pulled Pork

Serves 6
Ⓧ

Nutritional information per serving
276 Kcals
8.2g fat
11g net carbohydrates
37g protein

Ingredients
1kg pork shoulder, fat and skin removed (reserve to make pork crackling!)

300ml hot bone, pork or chicken broth

2 garlic cloves

50ml apple cider vinegar

50ml brandy or whisky

1 tbsp smoked paprika

1 tsp ground allspice

1 tsp mustard powder

1 tbsp mild chilli powder

1 tsp dried marjoram

1 tsp dried thyme

½ tsp ground ginger

½ tsp ground cinnamon

salt and black pepper, to taste

3 tbsp fibre syrup (erythritol-based)

2 tbsp sugar-free ketchup

Preheat your slow cooker, following the manufacturer's instructions.

Place the pork shoulder in the base of your slow cooker.

Mix the remaining ingredients until well combined and pour over the pork.

Set the slow cooker to Low and cook for 8–10 hours.

When you are ready to serve, remove the pork and, using two forks, pull the pork apart to create the pulled pork. You can return the pulled pork to the slow cooker to mix with the remaining sauce, if liked.

If you have never cooked with fennel, I urge you to try it. It goes beautifully with pork and gives a delicious, subtle, aniseedy flavour. This recipe is low in carbs but packed with healthy fat and protein, perfect for the keto way of eating.

Pork and Fennel Casserole

Serves 4
❄ ⊘

Nutritional information per serving
456 Kcals
32.7g fat
3.7g net carbohydrates
36.7g protein

Ingredients
1 tsp olive or coconut oil

500g boneless pork shoulder, diced

1 onion, diced

2 garlic cloves, crushed

1 fennel bulb, thinly sliced

1 tsp dried rosemary

2 tsp dried oregano

1 tsp dried thyme

350ml hot bone, chicken or pork broth

salt and black pepper, to taste

Preheat your slow cooker, following the manufacturer's instructions.

If your slow cooker has a sauté option, you can use this; if not, use a sauté pan on your hob. Heat the olive or coconut oil, add the pork and cook until brown, sealing in the flavour. Transfer to the slow cooker.

Add all the remaining ingredients, set to Low and cook for 6–8 hours.

Serve with celeriac mash and steamed green vegetables.

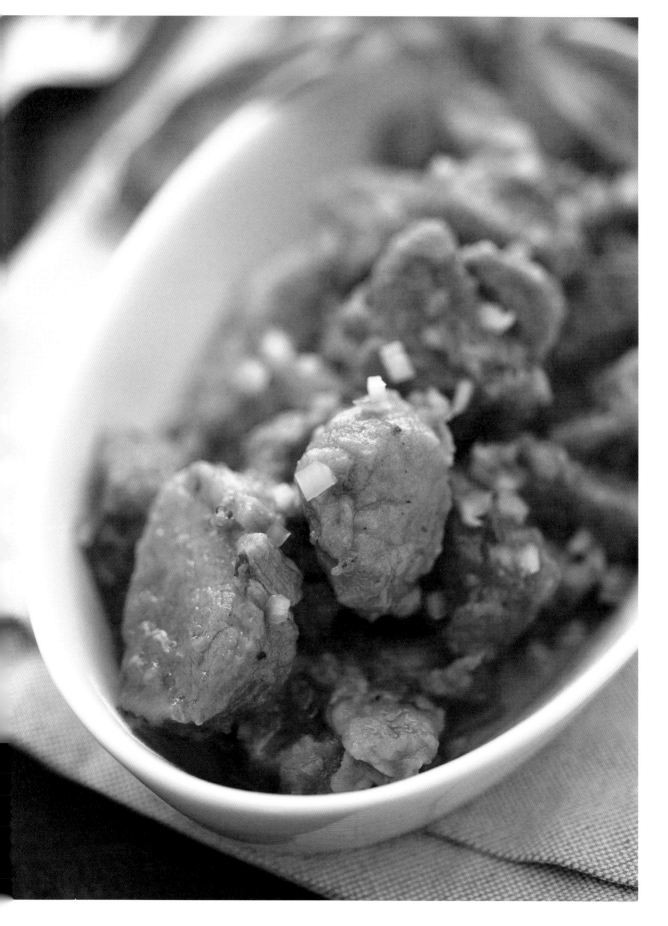

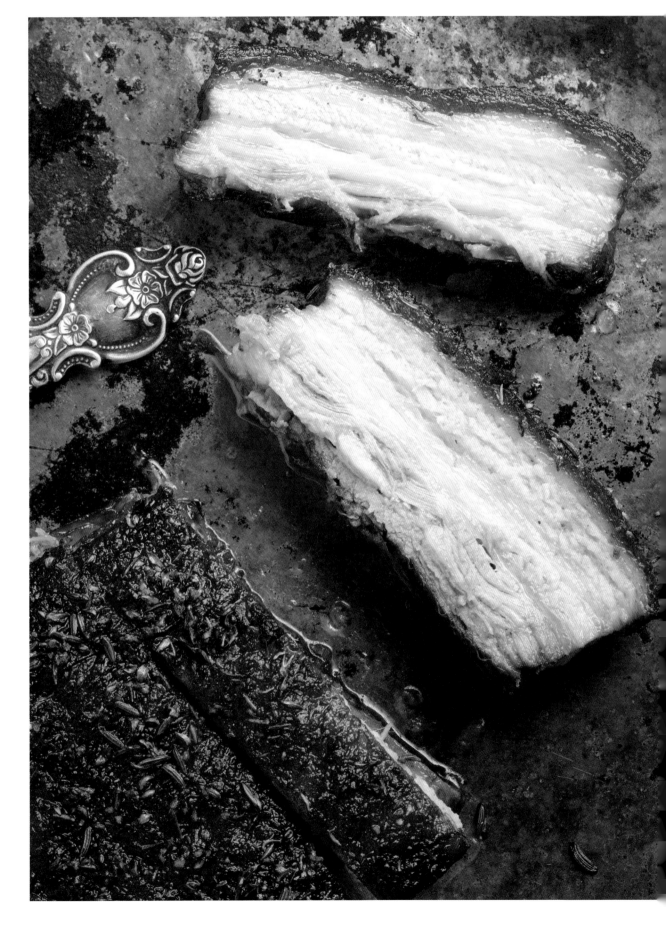

This is an easy way to cook a simple pork belly, ready to serve with some steamed vegetables or whatever you choose. It is a two-step process as it is so much nicer finished in the oven or on the hob before serving.

Slow-cooked Pork Belly

Serves 6

Nutritional information per serving
461 Kcals
34g fat
4.2g net carbohydrates
34g protein

Ingredients
2 onions, sliced

2 garlic cloves, crushed

3cm piece of fresh ginger, chopped

1kg pork belly

300ml hot bone broth

salt and black pepper, to taste

Preheat your slow cooker, following the manufacturer's instructions.

Arrange the sliced onion in the base of your slow cooker. Rub the garlic and ginger over the pork.

Place the pork belly on top of the onions and season to taste.

Pour the hot bone broth into the side of the slow cooker, being careful not to pour it over the pork.

Set to Low and cook for 6–8 hours.

Thirty minutes before you are ready to serve preheat the oven to 200°C (180°C fan) Gas 6.

Remove the pork belly from the slow cooker and transfer to a non-stick baking tray, then roast in the oven for 20 minutes until the skin has browned.

Serve immediately.

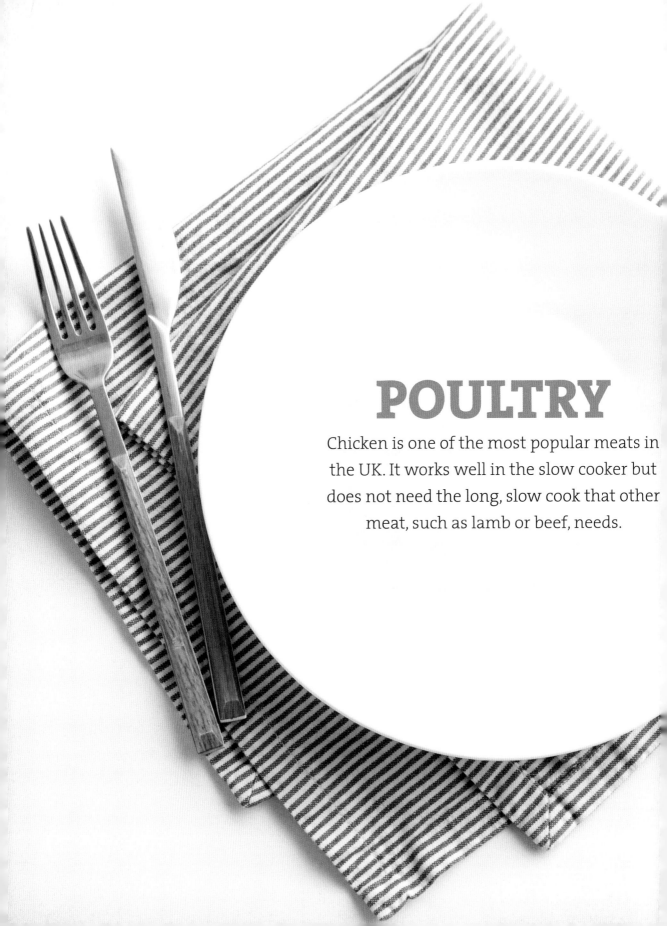

POULTRY

Chicken is one of the most popular meats in the UK. It works well in the slow cooker but does not need the long, slow cook that other meat, such as lamb or beef, needs.

Most families opt for chicken breast but I would recommend using thighs and leg meat as these are much more suited to longer cooks; the added bonus is that these are often much cheaper to buy and have more flavour. You can buy skinless and boneless chickens thighs, although why anyone would want to waste that delicious flavour and fat that's so vital for the ketogenic way of eating is beyond me!

Don't forget to save your bones if you are cooking a roast chicken. It makes an excellent and very nourishing chicken broth – see page 165 for the recipe.

BUTTERFLYING CHICKEN

You will need to butterfly chicken breasts for the stuffed chicken recipe. You can, of course, ask your butcher to do this for you, but it is actually very simple. There is also a recipe for stuffed turkey breast in this chapter – the technique for butterflying a turkey breast is the same, just on a larger scale.

1   Place your hand over the breast and using a very sharp knife carefully cut into it horizontally, but do not cut completely – you must stop before you reach the edge as you want it to open like butterfly wings or the pages of a book.

2   Cover with clingfilm and use a wooden kitchen mallet or rolling pin to bash lightly until you have a flat, butterfly-shaped chicken. This makes it much easier if you want to stuff and roll the chicken.

3   Once stuffed and rolled, you can hold it together with a wooden cocktail stick.

CREATING A CHICKEN POCKET

Another option if you want to stuff chicken is to create a pocket. This is great if you want to stuff with a few slices of mozzarella or similar.

1   Use a very sharp knife and cut a 4–5cm slit into the thickest part of the chicken breast. Make sure you do not cut all the way through.

2   Once you have stuffed the chicken you can hold it together with a wooden cocktail stick to stop the stuffing coming out.

If you like your curries with a bit of a kick, this one is for you; however, you can adjust the spices to suit your own palate. I love this with broccoli rice and a dollop of raita (natural yoghurt, cucumber and fresh mint). If you want a creamier base, add some coconut cream instead of the bone/chicken broth – this will also help mellow the heat.

Chicken Madras

Serves 6

❄ ⊘

Nutritional information per serving
235 Kcals
7.2g fat
7.7g net carbohydrates
33g protein

Ingredients
2 tbsp olive oil

2–3 red chillies, deseeded

3 garlic cloves

1 tbsp garam masala

½ tsp ground cinnamon

1 tsp ground coriander

1 tsp ground turmeric

1 tsp ground cumin

3 tomatoes

3cm piece of fresh ginger

1 tbsp tomato purée

a small handful of coriander leaves

1 large red onion, diced

750g boneless chicken, diced (breast, leg or thigh)

250ml hot bone or chicken broth (or use coconut cream, if preferred)

Put all the ingredients apart from the onion, chicken and broth into a food processor and whizz until you a paste forms.

If you are marinating the meat, place the chicken in a bowl or freezer bag, pour over the paste and turn to coat the chicken in the marinade. Leave for a few hours (you can skip this step if you don't have time).

Preheat your slow cooker, following the manufacturer's instructions.

Put the chicken, paste and diced onion into the slow cooker and stir to combine. Add the broth or coconut cream if you prefer a creamier base.

Set to Low and cook for 6 hours.

Serve with cauliflower or broccoli rice.

Top Tip
I like to marinate this for at least 2 hours before placing in the slow cooker. You don't have to do this, but I think it definitely improves the flavour.

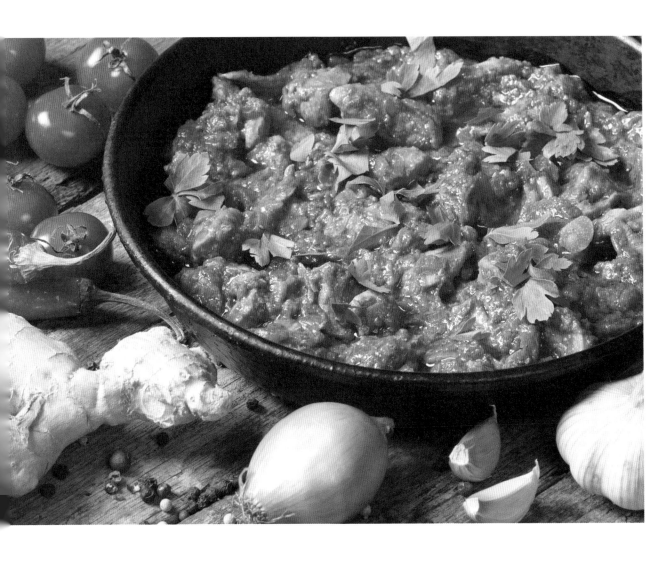

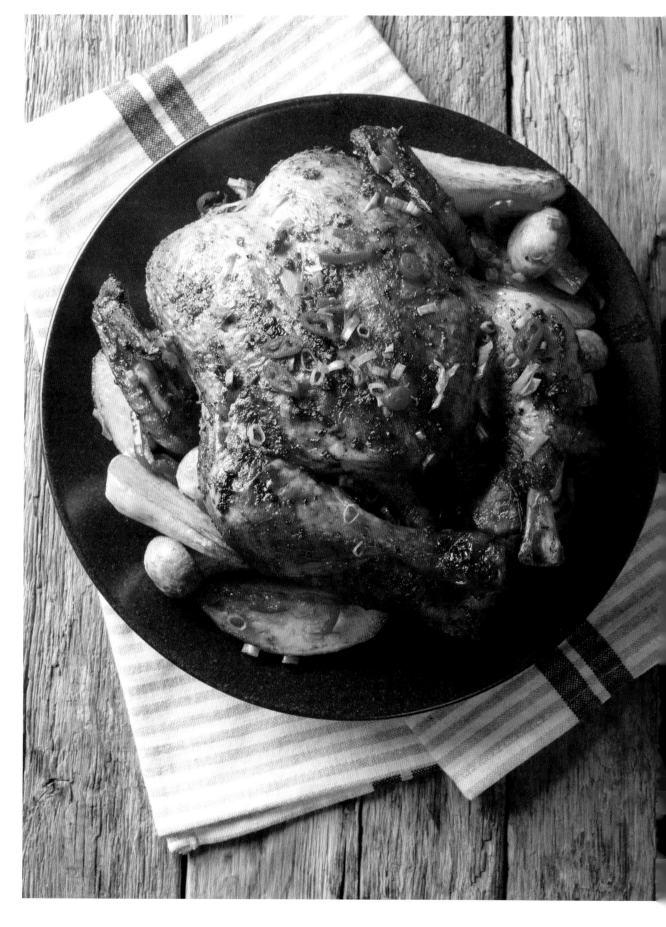

Slow-cooked whole chicken is incredibly tender and moist; it's one of my favourite ways to cook chicken. I coat the chicken generously with my harissa paste (see page 169) before placing into the slow cooker. It won't colour like oven-roasted chicken, so you may want to pop into a hot oven for the last 10–15 minutes in order to give it some colour. It sounds obvious but make sure your chicken fits in your slow cooker!

Slow-cooked Harissa Chicken

Serves 4–6

Ⓧ

Nutritional information per serving
354 Kcals
23g fat
4.8g net carbohydrates
30g protein

Ingredients
1 medium whole chicken (about 1.25kg)

4–5 tbsp Spiced Harissa Paste (see page 169)

1 onion, roughly chopped

250ml hot bone or chicken broth

salt and black pepper, to taste

Preheat the slow cooker, following the manufacturer's instructions.

Rub the chicken with a generous, even layer of my harissa paste – you may want to wear gloves for this as the paste contains a lot of chilli!

Arrange the sliced onion over the base of the slow cooker before adding the chicken.

Pour the hot chicken broth to the side of the chicken, carefully avoiding the harissa paste as you do not want to rinse it all off!

Set to Low and cook for 6 hours. Check the chicken is cooked by cutting into the gap between the leg and the breast; if the juices run clear it is done. If it needs a little longer, you can turn up to High and cook for another 30 minutes before checking again. The timings will depend on the size of the chicken used.

When you are ready to serve, place the chicken on a serving dish. Serve with celeriac chips (see page 151), buttered mushrooms and salad.

There is nothing more delicious than the flavours of the Mediterranean; I love the mixture of olives, sweet peppers, garlic, chorizo and oregano. This dish is lovely any time of the year – I serve it in the summer with a nice green salad and in the winter months with some cauliflower rice, or if I want real comfort food, I may make some cheesy cauliflower mash.

Spanish Chicken

Serves 4–6

❄ ⊘

Nutritional information per serving (calculated on 4 servings)
751 Kcals
55g fat
8g net carbohydrates
53g protein

Ingredients
1 tsp olive or coconut oil

4–6 skinless and boneless chicken thighs

225g chorizo, thickly sliced

1 red onion, sliced

2 garlic cloves, crushed

1 red pepper, deseeded and sliced

80g pitted black olives

2 tbsp sun-dried tomato purée

2 tsp dried oregano

1 tsp hot paprika

½ tsp cayenne pepper

½ tsp ground cinnamon

400ml hot bone or chicken broth

150g button mushrooms, halved

a small handful of fresh basil leaves, to garnish

Preheat your slow cooker, following the manufacturer's instructions.

If your slow cooker has a sauté function, use this to heat the oil and brown the chicken and chorizo; if not, use a sauté pan on your hob.

Transfer to the slow cooker and add all the remaining ingredients except the mushrooms and basil. Combine well to make sure everything is evenly distributed. Set to Low and cook for 6 hours. Half an hour before serving, add the mushrooms, switch to the High setting and cook for 30 minutes.

Garnish with basil leaves and serve with cauliflower rice, cauliflower mash or a green salad.

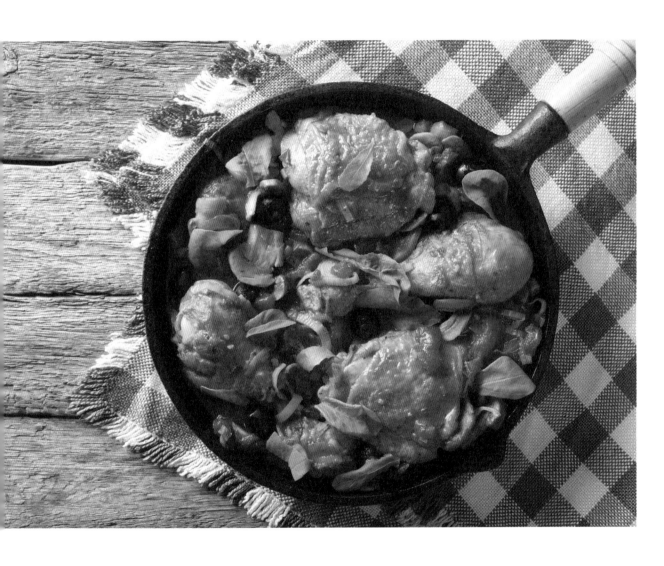

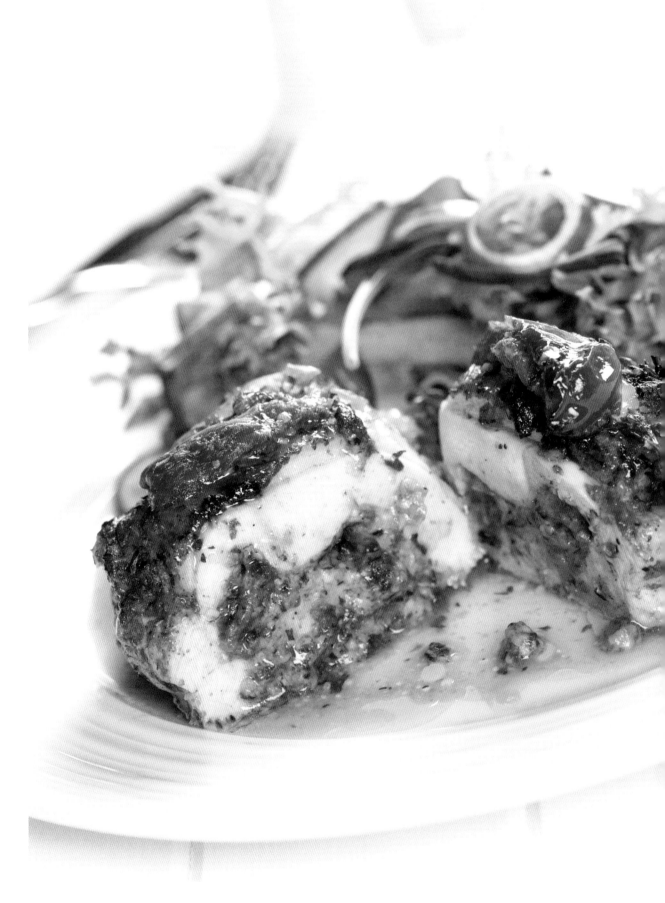

This is a massive hit in our home. I love the flavours of mozzarella with sun-dried tomatoes. This is a dish that can be made in advance – simply keep in the fridge until needed. If you prefer, you can wrap each breast with bacon. This will increase the calories, fat and protein but will not affect the carbohydrate count.

Italian Stuffed Chicken

Serves 4

Nutritional
information per
serving
335 Kcals
15g fat
1.1g net carbohydrates
47g protein

Ingredients
4 chicken breasts (about
800g total weight)

200g mozzarella cheese

30g sun-dried tomatoes,
plus extra, chopped, for
topping (optional)

2 tsp dried oregano

8 pitted green olives

1 tbsp capers

2 garlic cloves

a small handful of fresh
basil

300ml hot bone or
chicken broth (or use
white wine)

Preheat your slow cooker, following the manufacturer's instructions.

Butterfly each chicken breast using a very sharp knife (see page 87). Open it up; if it is uneven, just bash a little with a wooden rolling pin until it forms a flat butterfly ready for you to stuff and roll.

Put the mozzarella, sun-dried tomatoes, oregano, olives, capers, garlic and basil into a food processor and pulse very lightly until it is just mixed. Do not over process – you want a nice mix, but not a paste. If you don't have a processor, simply chop the ingredients into small pieces and mix well.

Spread a generous spoonful of the mixture down the middle of each chicken breast and carefully roll up to form a parcel – use a wooden cocktail stick to secure, if you like. Place the stuffed breasts seam down into the slow cooker.

Pour the chicken broth into the slow cooker and scatter over the extra chopped sun-dried tomatoes (if using) and any remaining mozzarella mixture.

Set to Low and cook for 3–4 hours until cooked through.

Serve with a drizzle of the broth poured over and a delicious salad on the side.

This is my version of Manchurian, a Chinese–Indian fusion of flavours. Traditionally this is made with minced chicken, shaped into balls and fried in a batter before being coated in the Manchurian sauce, but I have given it a keto twist, while retaining the same delicious flavour. This is lovely on its own, but you can of course serve with some cauliflower rice.

Manchurian-style Chicken

Serves 4

Ⓧ

Nutritional information per serving
291 Kcals
5.6g fat
7.5g net carbohydrates
50g protein

Ingredients
750g boneless chicken (thigh or breast), diced

1 small red onion, thinly sliced

1 red and 1 yellow pepper, deseeded and diced

300ml hot bone or chicken broth

3 garlic cloves, crushed

4cm piece of fresh ginger, grated

2 chillies, finely chopped

½ tsp chilli powder

½ tsp paprika

1 tbsp smooth almond butter

2 tbsp Kikkoman gluten-free soy sauce

1 tbsp tomato purée

salt and black pepper, to taste

2 spring onions, thinly sliced, to garnish

Preheat your slow cooker, following the manufacturer's instructions.

Put the chicken, onion and peppers into the slow cooker. In a jug mix the broth with all the remaining ingredients except the spring onions. Season to taste.

Combine well before pouring over the chicken and vegetables.

Set to Low and cook for 6 hours.

Serve garnished with sliced spring onions.

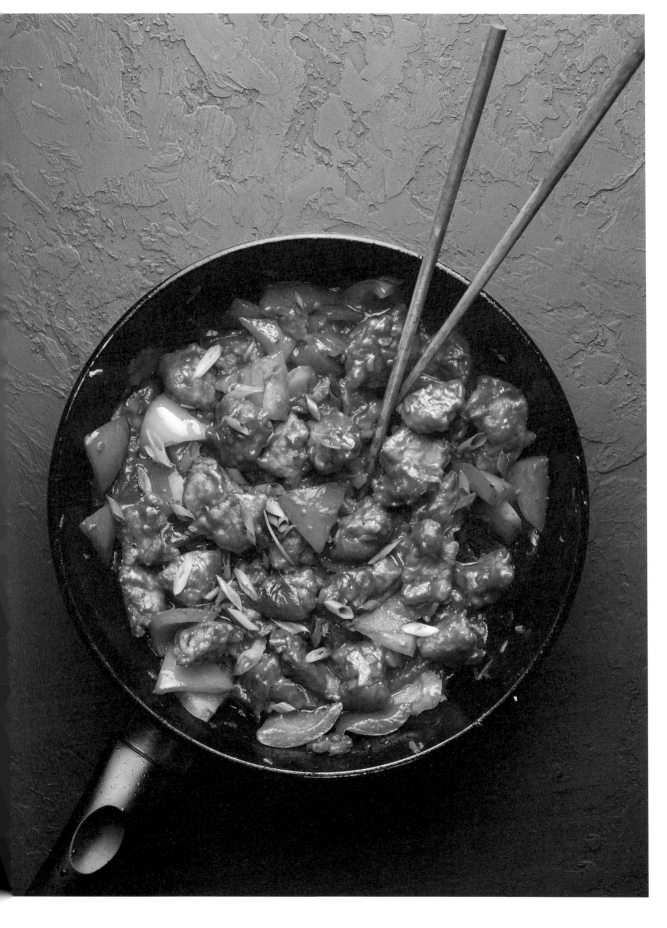

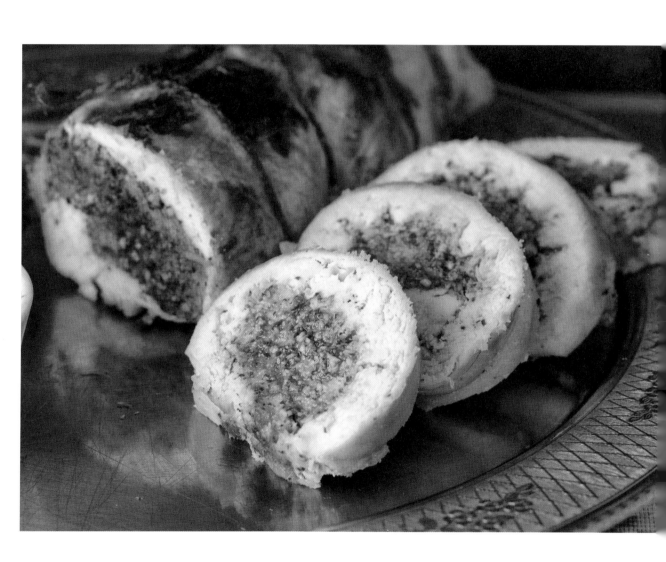

Turkey is a great meat but tends to be a little dry at times. The slow cooker is a fantastic way to cook turkey as it keeps the meat nice and moist. If you want to add a little more flavour, you can cover the breast with pancetta or bacon rashers, though these won't brown in the slow cooker so will need to be finished in the oven or under the grill in order to get the nice crisp, golden finish. This recipe uses my delicious Chilli and Coriander Pesto (page 173).

Coriander and Chilli Stuffed Turkey Breast

Serves 6

Nutritional information per serving
264 Kcals
8.2g fat
2.3g net carbohydrates
44g protein

You will need
Kitchen twine/string

Ingredients
1kg boneless turkey breast, butterflied (see page 87)

4–5 tbsp chilli and coriander pesto (see page 173)

1 onion, thickly sliced

500ml hot bone or chicken broth

Preheat your slow cooker, following the manufacturer's instructions.

Open out the butterflied turkey breast and score the flesh well with a sharp knife.

Cover with clingfilm and use a wooden mallet or rolling pin to bash the turkey breast until it is level – this is also a great way to relieve any stress! Trim the edges if you need to; the aim is to get as close as possible to a rectangle shape in order to be able to roll up the turkey breast easily.

Once you have the thickness and shape you are happy with, spread generously with the chilli and coriander pesto.

Carefully roll up the turkey breast as tight as you can to form a log shape. Tie tightly with string, 3 or 4 times along the log, to hold it all together.

Arrange the onion slices in the base of the slow cooker. Sit the turkey log on top before adding the broth.

Set to Low and cook for 4–5 hours until cooked through.

Remove from the slow cooker. You can use the broth to make a gravy if you wish.

Remove the string and cut into thick slices before serving.

I love spicy curries but some prefer a creamier, mellow flavour so this is the perfect recipe for them. It works well in the slow cooker as it allow the flavours to melt into the chicken. I like to double up all my curry recipes and store in 1–2 portion sizes in the freezer, ready to pull out a variety to make the perfect, effortless curry night. Serve with broccoli or cauliflower mash.

Creamy Chicken Korma

Serves 4–6
❄ ⊘

Nutritional information per serving
413 Kcals
21g fat
8.4g net carbohydrates
47g protein

Ingredients
2 garlic cloves

3cm piece of fresh ginger

1 red chilli, deseeded

2 tsp ground cumin

2 tsp ground coriander

1 tsp ground turmeric

salt and black pepper, to taste

1 tbsp tomato purée

400g full-fat coconut milk

750g skinless and boneless chicken (breast or thigh), cut into large chunks

1 onion, diced

chopped coriander leaves, to garnish

Preheat your slow cooker, following the manufacturer's instructions.

Put the garlic, ginger, chilli, cumin, coriander and turmeric into a food processor with some salt and pepper. Add the tomato purée and coconut milk and whizz until smooth.

Put the chicken and the onion into the slow cooker, add the korma sauce and mix to combine.

Set to Low and cook for 5–6 hours.

Serve garnished with the chopped coriander leaves.

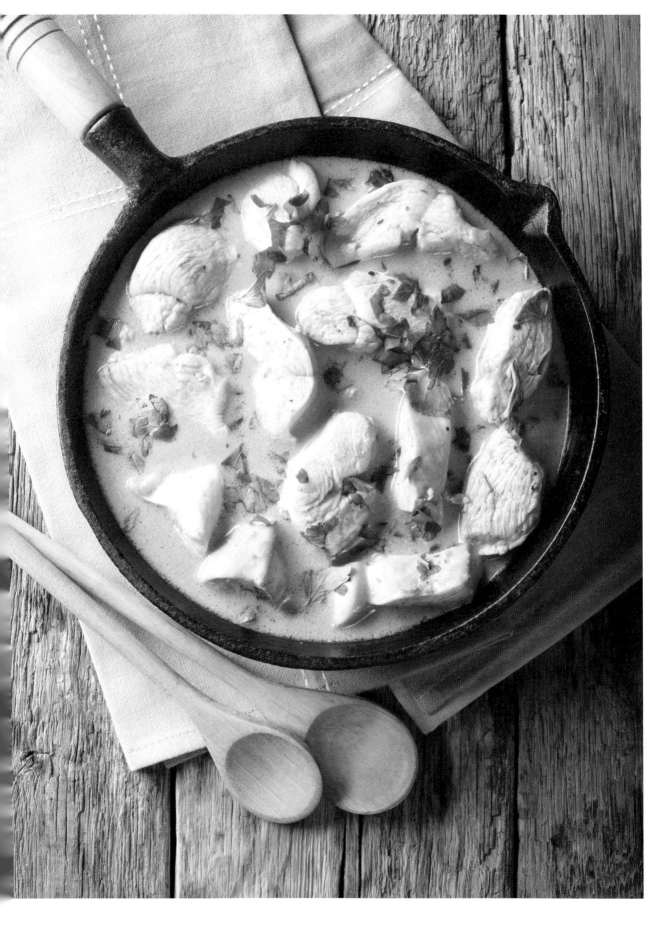

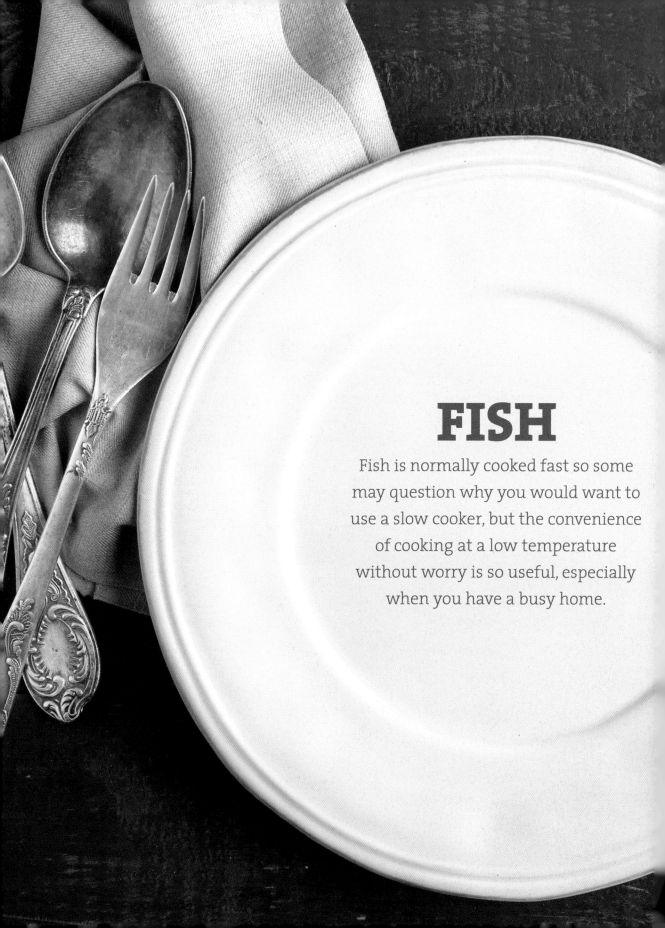

FISH

Fish is normally cooked fast so some may question why you would want to use a slow cooker, but the convenience of cooking at a low temperature without worry is so useful, especially when you have a busy home.

You may be surprised at what you can do in the slow cooker and how delicious the fish can taste when cooked this way. It also traps the odours, so your kitchen doesn't become overpowered with the smell of fish when cooking. You may want to adapt your own recipes to suit or try something new based on this advice. Speak to your fishmonger to discuss the right type of fish for the slow cooker.

Cooking fish in the slow cooker can really enhance the flavour, however, you will have to consider cooking times. We are so used to slow cookers fitting around our busy lives, but fish recipes might not be so accommodating. Fish does not need long cooking times so you will be looking at a maximum of 3–4 hours and it needs to be eaten straight away as it will dry out if left on warm. This may be less appealing if you want to prepare your slow cooker to cook all day while you are at work.

POACHING
Poaching fish only takes about 45 minutes on high. Add your fish with the stock or water and simply poach with a few herbs to add flavour.

SHELLFISH
If you like shellfish, add them towards the end of the cooking time otherwise they may spoil. If cooking on High, this can be in the last 20 minutes. If you are using frozen shellfish, make sure they are defrosted completely before adding to the slow cooker.

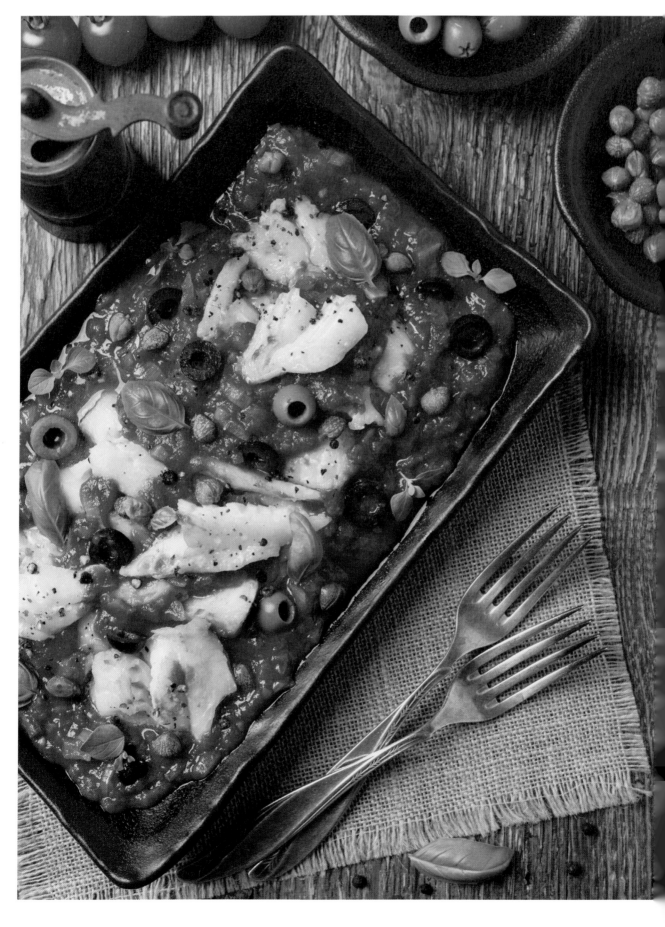

If you love the Mediterranean flavours of tomato, garlic, olives and basil, you will love this dish. I have thrown in some chorizo as I love the smoky flavour, but you can swap this for some diced smoked pancetta if you prefer. This dish can be served on its own with a lovely green salad or, for a more filling meal, some spiralised courgette.

Mediterranean Cod

Serves 4

Nutritional information per serving
320 Kcals
16g fat
8.8g net carbohydrates
33g protein

Ingredients
150g chorizo, diced

1 onion, finely chopped

2 garlic cloves, crushed

1 red pepper, deseeded and diced

400g tin chopped tomatoes

½ tbsp red wine vinegar

1 tsp dried tarragon

½ tsp dried basil

1 tsp dried oregano

1 tsp dried parsley

10 pitted black olives, sliced

8 pitted green olives, halved

1 tbsp capers

4 cod fillets (about 500g total weight)

salt and black pepper, to taste

Preheat your slow cooker, following the manufacturer's instructions.

Put the chorizo into the slow cooker on the sauté setting. (If you don't have a sauté function, use a sauté pan on the hob and then transfer to the slow cooker.) Cook the chorizo for 5 minutes until the flavours and oils start to release.

Put all the remaining ingredients into the slow cooker apart from the olives, capers and cod. Season to taste before combining well.

Set to High and cook for 2 hours.

Add the olives, capers and cod fillets and cook for another 30 minutes– 1 hour, depending on the thickness of the cod fillets. The fish should be nice and flaky when cooked.

Serve with a salad or spiralised courgette.

Eggs are one of the best foods for the ketogenic way of eating and frittatas are so easy and delicious. I am always trying to promote more oily fish in my clients' diets, and nothing is better than eating plenty of salmon. This is a simple yet delicious frittata combining salmon and Camembert for a creamy, omega-3 rich meal. Perfect for a light lunch or simple dinner served with a delicious salad.

Salmon and Camembert Frittata

Serves 6

Nutritional information per serving
458 Kcals
38g fat
2.5g net carbohydrates
25g protein

Ingredients
butter or olive oil, for greasing
1 onion, finely chopped
2 salmon fillets (about 250g total weight), chopped
grated zest of ½ lemon
200g Camembert, sliced
6 eggs
200ml double cream
a few sprigs of fresh dill, finely chopped
black pepper, to taste

Preheat your slow cooker, following the manufacturer's instructions.

Grease the base of the slow cooker well with butter or olive oil. If you are nervous about it sticking, you could line with baking parchment or use a large cake liner.

Place the onion and salmon in the base of the slow cooker. Squeeze some lemon juice over the salmon to taste.

Add the camembert slices.

Beat the eggs and cream together, add the dill and season with pepper. Pour this over the salmon. It will soak through ensuring the whole thing is covered.

Set to High and cook for 1–2 hours.

When cooked, remove the pot from the cooker base. Run a sharp knife around the edge to help loosen the frittata. Carefully place a plate over the pot and invert so the frittata drops on to the plate.

Serve hot or cold with salad.

If you don't like too much heat, this dish is perfect for you. Simple to prepare and full of omega-3 fats, this dish really hits the spot when you are in need of some comfort food. As with all my curries, serve with cauliflower rice.

Salmon in Creamy Thai Red Sauce

Serves 4

Nutritional information per serving
583 Kcals
46g fat
7.6g net carbohydrates
34g protein

Ingredients
2–3 tbsp Thai Red Curry Paste (see page 178)

1 tbsp smooth almond butter

400g tin full-fat coconut milk

1 tbsp fish sauce (optional)

1 onion, finely chopped

4 fresh salmon fillets

2 spring onions, thinly sliced

a small handful of fresh coriander leaves

Preheat your slow cooker, following the manufacturer's instructions.

Mix the curry paste with the almond butter, coconut milk and fish sauce (if using), making sure it is smooth and lump-free.

Put the onion and salmon fillets into the slow cooker and pour over the coconut milk mixture.

Set to High and cook for 1–1½ hours until the salmon is cooked (the cooking time will depend on the thickness of the salmon).

Serve the salmon, drizzled in the sauce, with a side of cauliflower rice. Garnish with sliced spring onions and some coriander leaves.

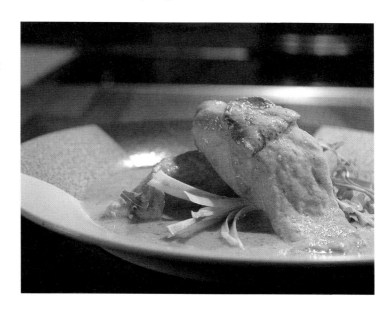

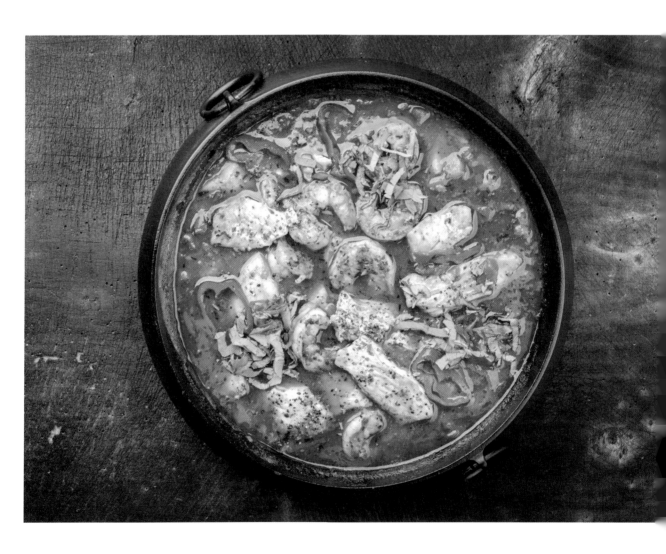

This is a really tasty fish stew, with a rich, spicy stock. It is wonderfully filling and packed with omega-3 fats. I have opted for a very simple fish selection in this dish, but you can add whatever fish fillets or seafood you prefer. Speak to your fishmonger for recommendations.

Hot and Spicy Fish Gumbo

Serves 4
⊘

Nutritional information per serving
370 Kcals
20g fat
8.3g net carbohydrates
37g protein

Ingredients
2 tsp olive oil

1 onion, finely chopped

1 large red pepper, deseeded and finely chopped

3 garlic cloves, crushed

2 red chillies, deseeded and finely chopped

200g chorizo, sliced or diced

400g tin chopped tomatoes

2 tsp tomato purée

350ml fish stock

1 tbsp fish sauce (optional)

1 tsp dried parsley

2 tsp smoked paprika

1 tsp onion powder

¼ tsp cayenne pepper

2 tsp dried oregano

1 tsp ground coriander

300g salmon fillets, diced

250g white cod fillet, diced

250g prawns (defrosted if frozen), deveined and peeled

a small handful of fresh parsley leaves

a small handful of fresh coriander leaves

Preheat your slow cooker, following the manufacturer's instructions.

In a sauté pan (or use the sauté function if your slow cooker has this) heat the olive oil and add the onion, pepper, garlic, chillies and chorizo. Cook for 5–8 minutes until lightly softened.

Transfer to the slow cooker with the chopped tomatoes, tomato purée, fish stock, fish sauce (if using) and herbs and spices.

Add the fish fillets, set to High and cook for 1–2 hours (or 2–4 hours on Low).

Add the prawns, fresh parsley and coriander and cook on High for a further 30 minutes.

Serve with cauliflower rice.

Salmon usually has subtle flavours added to it, but this dish packs a punch using my homemade spiced harissa paste. It is delicious with cauliflower rice and a green salad. You can prepare the salmon in advance and keep the parcels in the fridge until you are ready to cook.

Harissa Salmon

Serves 4

Nutritional information per serving
396 Kcals
29g fat
1.3g net carbohydrates
31g protein

Ingredients
4 salmon fillets (about 150g each)

4 heaped tsp Spiced Harissa Paste (see page 169)

salt and black pepper, to taste

4 tsp olive oil

Preheat your slow cooker, following the manufacturer's instructions.

Place 4 squares of foil on your worktop, large enough to wrap each salmon fillet (alternatively, you can cook all the salmon fillets in one parcel).

Place a salmon fillet into the centre of each piece of foil. Spread the harissa paste over the top (it is easier to do this on the foil as it creates less mess). Repeat with the other salmon fillets.

Season thoroughly before adding a small drizzle of olive oil, roughly 1 teaspoon per fish.

Wrap the foil securely and place in the base of the slow cooker.

Pop on the lid, set to Low and cook for 2–3 hours. Cooking times will depend on the size and thickness of your salmon fillets. Take care when removing the salmon as the foil gets very hot.

Serve with cauliflower rice and green salad.

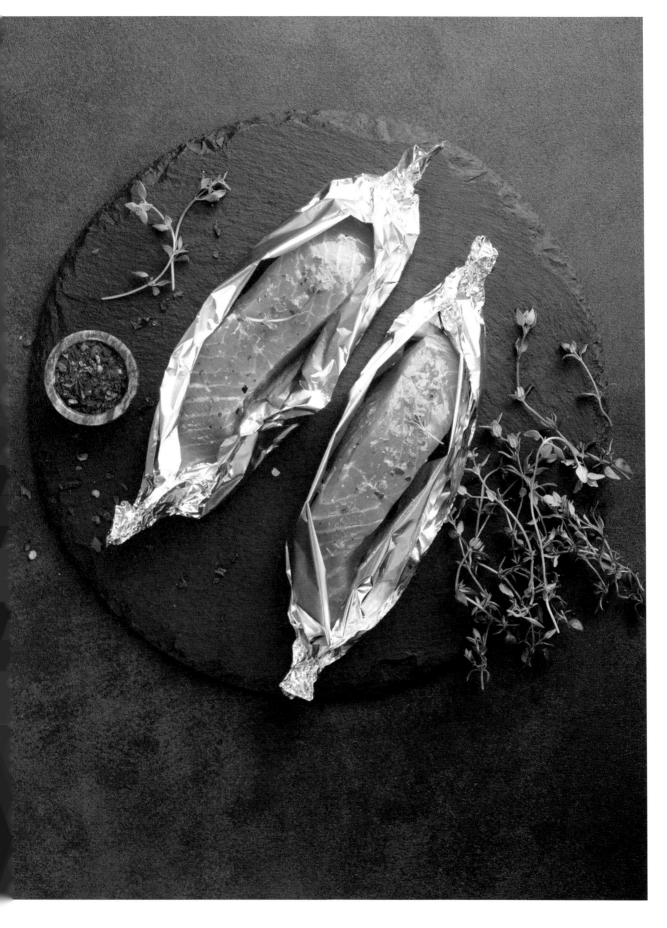

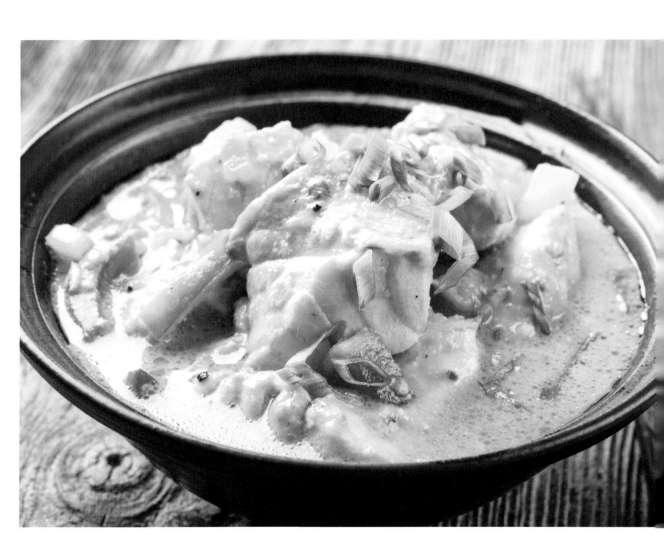

This is a wonderfully creamy fish curry with a Thai flavour, suitable for all the family as it is not too hot. You can of course adjust the heat by adding more chillies if you prefer more of a kick.

Thai Green Fish Curry

Serves 4

Nutritional information per serving
347 Kcals
22g fat
7.1g net carbohydrates
29g protein

Ingredients
4 spring onions, cut into 4–6cm lengths (including green leaves)

1 large red pepper, deseeded and diced

2 garlic cloves, roughly chopped

2cm piece of fresh ginger, finely chopped

grated zest and juice of ½ lime

4 tbsp Thai Green Curry Paste (see page 177)

1 tsp ground turmeric (poor man's saffron!)

400ml can coconut milk

600g white fish fillets, skinned and quartered (use cod, haddock or pollock)

Preheat your slow cooker, following the manufacturer's instructions.

Put all the ingredients, apart from the fish, into the slow cooker. Combine well.

Set to High and cook for 1 hour before adding the fish. Cook for a further 1–1½ hours until the fish is cooked to your taste (the cooking time will depend on the size and thickness of your fish).

Serve with cauliflower rice.

Fish pie is the ultimate comfort food. The creamy sauce combines well with the cheesy mash. This is a two-step process as you cook the base in the slow cooker before adding the cheesy cauliflower mash but don't let that put you off; it is a really tasty dish.

Keto Fish Pie

Serves 6

Nutritional information per serving
598 Kcals
50g fat
3.8g net carbohydrates
26.9g protein

Ingredients
500g mixed fish pieces (can buy fish pie mix)
500ml double cream
200g mature Cheddar, grated
½ tsp mustard powder
a small handful of fresh parsley
large head of cauliflower, broken into florets
50g butter
200g prawns
salt and black pepper, to taste

Preheat your slow cooker, following the manufacturer's recommendations.

Put the fish into the base of your slow cooker and season well.

Combine the cream, half the cheese, the mustard powder and parsley and pour this over the fish.

Set to Low and cook for 1 hour.

Meanwhile, prepare the topping. Steam the cauliflower florets until just soft then mash with the butter. Season well to taste before adding the remaining grated cheese. Combine well.

When the fish has had an hour in the slow cooker, add the prawns and combine well. Add the mash to the top of the fish base and smooth over, then continue to cook on Low for 30 minutes.

Before serving, if you want a golden topping, remove the base from the slow cooker and place it under a hot grill until golden.

Serve with steamed green vegetables.

Top Tip
For a variation on the cauliflower mash topping, trying using a mixture of cauliflower and broccoli. Alternatively, you can opt for a celeriac mash.

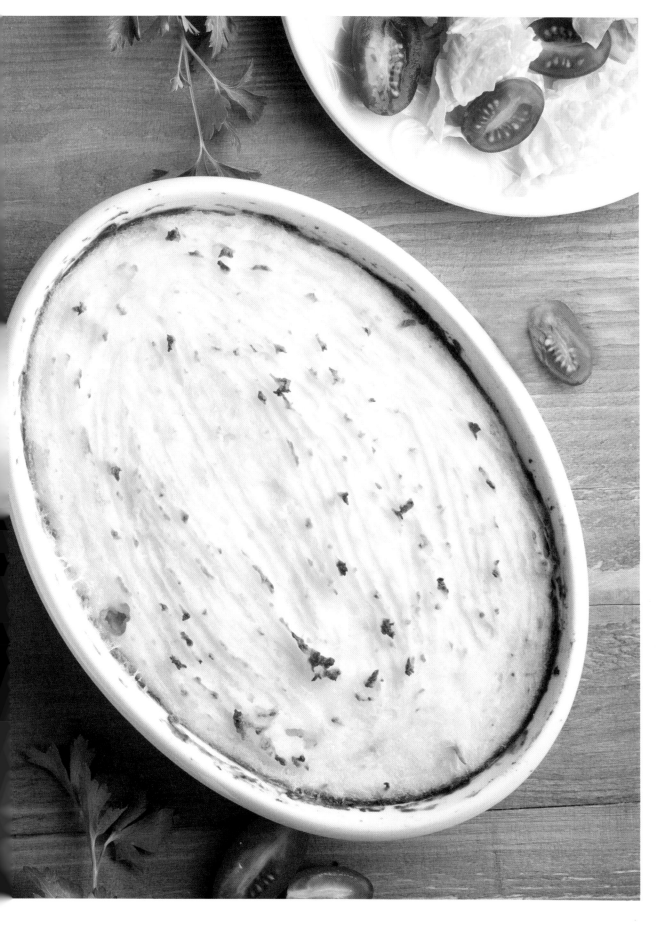

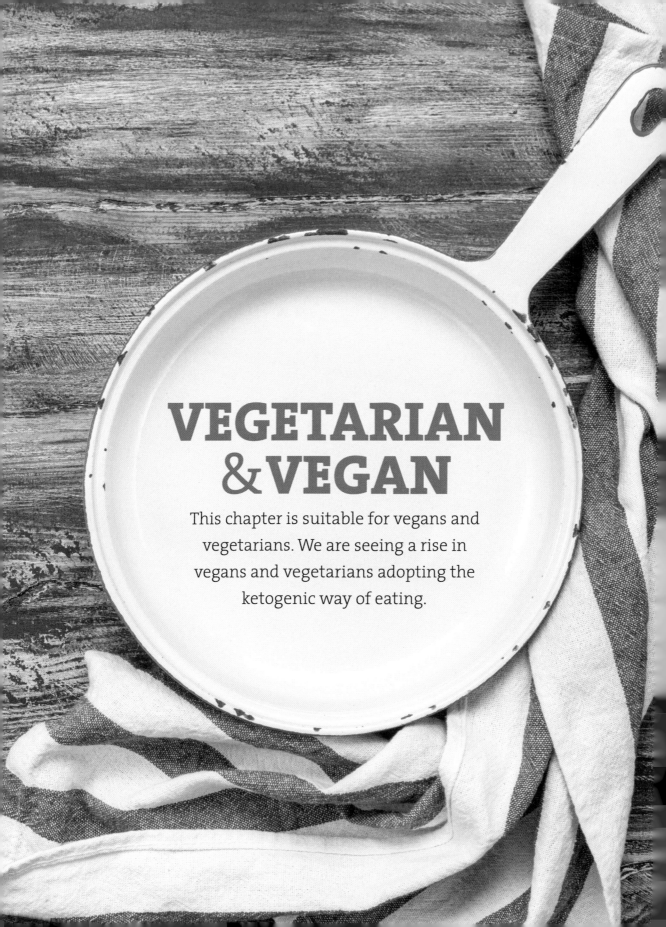

VEGETARIAN & VEGAN

This chapter is suitable for vegans and vegetarians. We are seeing a rise in vegans and vegetarians adopting the ketogenic way of eating.

Vegan and plant-based lifestyles are growing increasingly popular, but sadly this has resulted in a rise in 'fake' food. It is important when opting for a vegan way of eating, to ensure you have enough quality nutrients in your diet, in particular good protein, healthy fats, minerals, especially iron, and vitamins, especially B12. It is essential, therefore, that you get your food from natural sources that are nutrient-rich.

It is not as easy to follow a ketogenic way of eating when vegan. It takes a lot of planning and care. Many adapt their food lists to include more protein-based foods in order to achieve good nourishment and meet the macros. There are curds you can use as a protein source, such as paneer (which is made from cow's milk), tofu or tempeh. Nuts and seeds, including nut butter, is key to this way of eating. You can buy vegan faux dairy products, though I would be careful with these as most contain unhealthy and non-keto ingredients as well as lots of inflammatory oils. Some keto vegans include pulses in order to gain more nutrients, though I have not added these in this chapter. These recipes are all delicious and suitable for meat eaters as well as vegetarians.

I love curries and this is one of my personal favourites as it is light and has a nice sweetness. It is really a keto take on aloo gobi, but instead of using potato, I have diced some celeriac. You could try this with radishes too as these also give a potato-like effect. Curries freeze well – I like to batch cook my curries and place them in labelled containers in the freezer, ready to pull out for curry night.

Cauliflower Curry

Serves 4

🔖 ❄ ⊘

Nutritional information per serving
241 Kcals
16g fat
15g net carbohydrates
6.3g protein

Ingredients
2 tsp coconut oil

1 onion, finely chopped

2 garlic cloves, crushed

1–2 chillies, deseeded and chopped

3cm piece of fresh ginger, grated

1 tsp ground turmeric

1–2 tsp chilli powder

1 tsp fennel seeds, crushed

1 tsp cumin seeds, crushed

2 tsp coriander seeds, crushed

½ tsp mustard powder

400g tin chopped tomatoes

1 cauliflower, cut into small florets

200g celeriac, diced into small cubes

1 heaped tbsp soft smooth almond butter

200ml (½ tin) coconut milk

200ml vegetable broth (use bone broth if not vegan)

a handful of fresh coriander or parsley leaves, to garnish

Preheat your slow cooker, following the manufacturer's instructions.

Put the coconut oil, onion, garlic, chillies, ginger and spices into the slow cooker and set to sauté function. If your slow cooker does not have a sauté function, use a sauté pan on your hob and then transfer to the slow cooker. Cook for 2–4 minutes until the flavours start to release.

Add all the remaining ingredients to the slow cooker, adding only enough broth to just cover the vegetables. Set to Low and cook for 6–8 hours.

Scatter over some fresh coriander or parsley leaves before serving with broccoli or cauliflower rice.

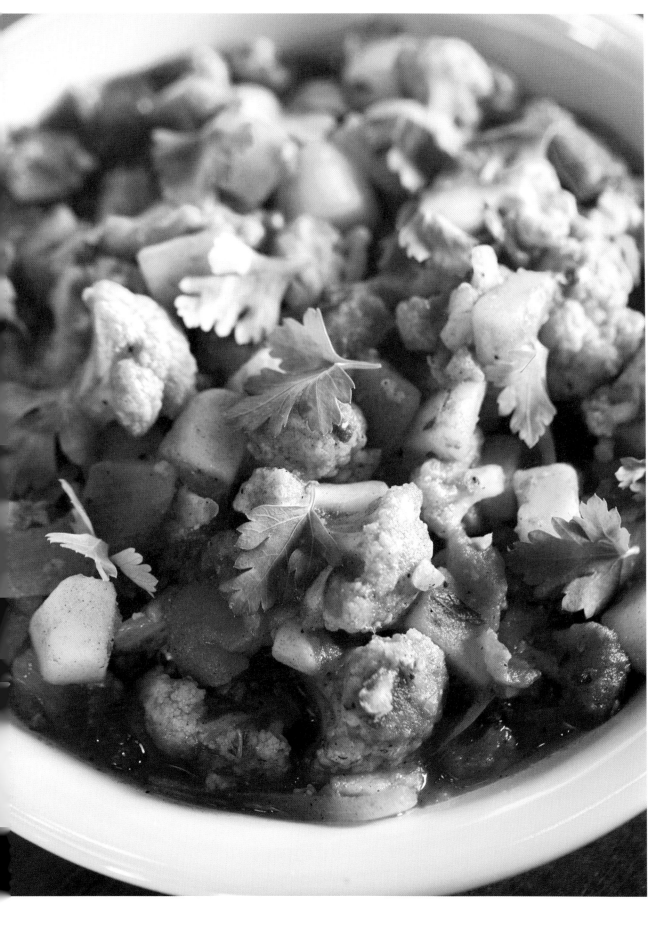

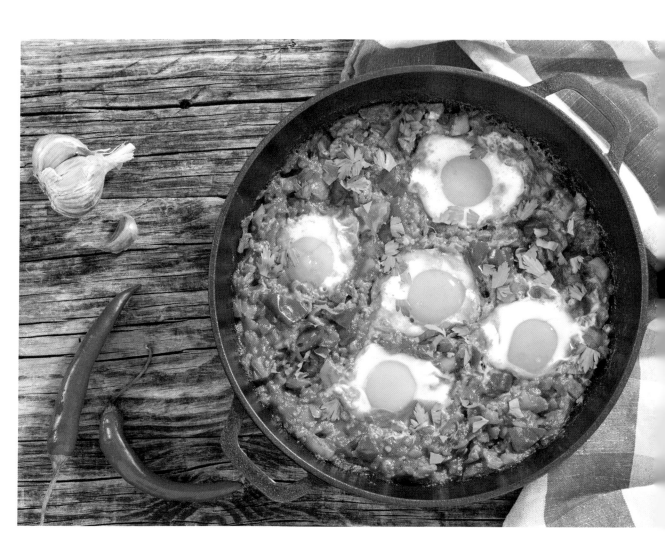

This has traditionally been a brunch dish, but I think it makes a wonderful meal. If you are not vegetarian, you could add some chopped smoked bacon or pancetta to the dish. I have kept this recipe quite mild with only one deseeded chilli added to the dish, but if you like things hot, feel free to add more to taste. This recipe is normally made in a sauté pan, but the slow cooker is brilliant as you can prep and leave the tomato sauce to cook and infuse over a few hours, adding the eggs 20–30 minutes before serving.

Loaded Shakshuka

Serves 4

Nutritional information per serving
240 Kcals
16g fat
8.7g net carbohydrates
13g protein

Ingredients
400g tin chopped tomatoes

1 small onion, finely chopped

2 garlic cloves, finely chopped

1 small red pepper, deseeded and diced

1 small yellow pepper, deseeded and diced

1–2 red chillies, deseeded and finely chopped, to taste

½ tsp smoked paprika

1 tsp ground cumin

1 tsp dried oregano

1 tsp dried parsley

2 tbsp sun-dried tomato purée

salt and black pepper, to taste

4 eggs

100g crumbled feta

Preheat your slow cooker, following the manufacturer's instructions.

Put all the ingredients into the slow cooker, apart from the eggs and feta. Season before combining well. If you are adding bacon or pancetta to the recipe, sauté this in a separate pan on the hob before adding to the slow cooker.

Set to High and cook for 1–2 hours until the sauce is cooked to your required softness (depends on how small you have diced the vegetables). If you have doubled up the sauce recipe, you can remove some now and allow to cool before storing in the fridge or freezer.

Crack one egg at a time into a cup or small jug. Try to make a little gap in the sauce – easier said than done if the sauce is quite loose! Tip the egg into the gap and repeat using up all the eggs. Sprinkle over half the crumbled feta.

Cook on High for another 8–20 minutes until your eggs are cooked to your liking – I like mine with a lovely runny yolk, so I aim for 8–12 minutes.

Serve immediately, with the remaining crumbled feta scattered over the top.

Note
Although the finished dish can't be frozen you can double up the sauce; simply remove half just before adding your eggs, cool and freeze this to use in a similar dish or even with pasta or as a topping for a keto pizza.

Eggs are a keto staple, and nothing is nicer than a crustless quiche when you fancy something tasty for lunch. This is one of my 'throw-it-all-in pies', where I use up my leftover vegetables and add what I fancy as and when. For the simplicity of this recipe, I am sticking to eggs, cheese and spinach, but feel free to add to suit any of your favourite ingredients, such as chopped ham, chorizo, mushrooms or leftover cooked veg.

Spinach and Cheese Crustless Quiche

Makes 8 slices

Nutritional information per slice
283 Kcals
26g fat
1.4g net carbohydrates
9.8g protein

Ingredients
butter, for greasing

1 small onion, finely chopped

80g baby leaf spinach

120g extra-mature Cheddar, grated

6 eggs, beaten

250ml double cream

1 tsp dried oregano

1 tsp dried parsley

salt and black pepper, to taste

Preheat your slow cooker, following the manufacturer's recommendations.

Ensure the slow cooker is very well greased. Alternatively, you can use a slow cooker liner, cake liner or line the slow cooker with baking parchment, which makes it easier to remove the quiche.

Scatter the onion into the base of your slow cooker. Top with the spinach and cheese.

Mix the eggs and cream together in a jug until combined well. Add the herbs and season well.

Pour into the slow cooker until everything is covered.

Set to High and cook for 1–2 hours or low for 3–4 hours until firm to touch.

Eat hot or cold.

Top Tip
If you fancy this for breakfast, you can prepare it in advance and plug your slow cooker into a timer to come on when needed.

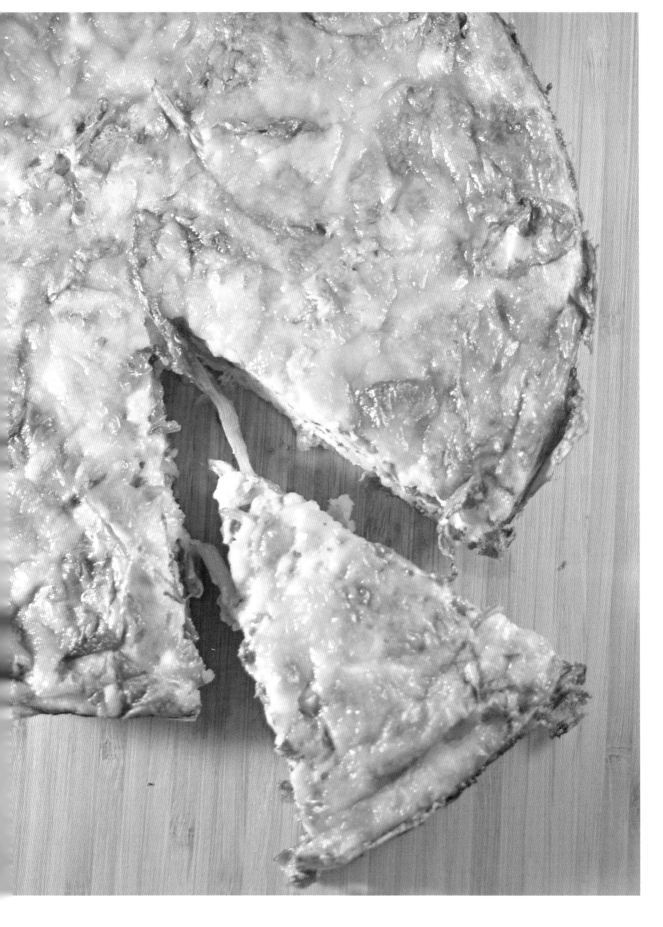

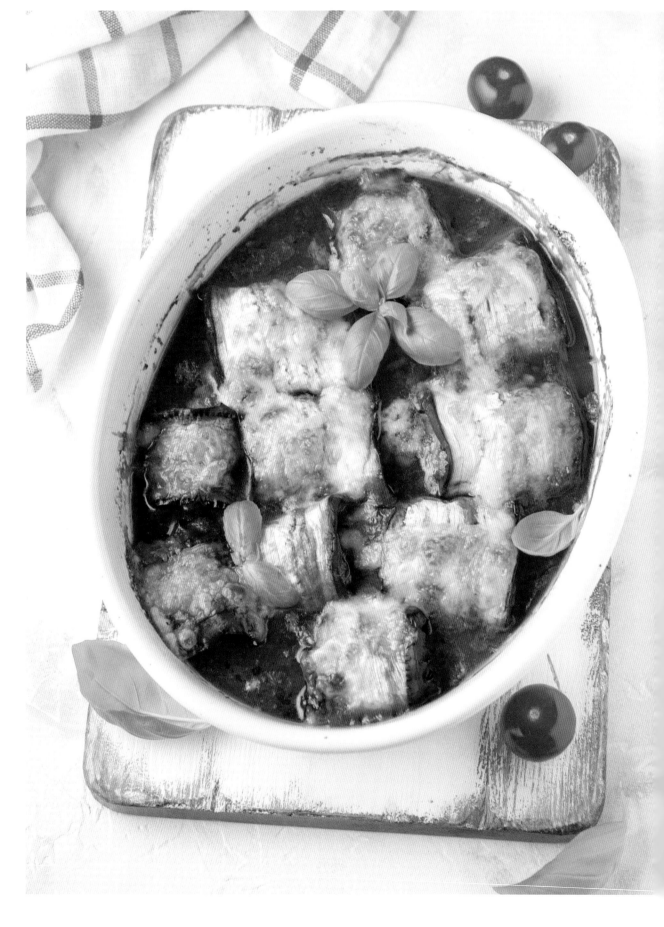

This is my variation of an Italian dish where you stuff aubergine slices with ricotta and serve in a delicious tomato sauce. You have to be very careful when you make these, allowing the aubergine rolls to cook without fiddling with them too much as they break apart easily. I would suggest finishing with a sprinkle of Parmesan or mature Cheddar and popping under the grill to brown before serving.

Slow-cooked Rollatini

Serves 4

Nutritional information per serving
348 Kcals
22g fat
8.8g net carbohydrates
27g protein

Ingredients
1 large aubergine

sea salt

400g tin chopped tomatoes

1 small onion, very finely chopped

2 garlic cloves, finely chopped

2 tsp dried oregano

½ tsp dried thyme

½ tsp dried basil

100ml vegetable broth (use bone broth if not vegetarian)

150g baby leaf spinach

250g mascarpone (or use coconut cream if dairy-free)

½ tsp grated nutmeg

50g grated Parmesan, mozzarella or mature Cheddar (leave out if dairy-free)

salt and black pepper, to taste

Preheat your slow cooker, following the manufacturer's instructions.

Slice the aubergine lengthways, as thinly as you can. Place the slices on a plate or baking tray lined with kitchen towel and sprinkle with sea salt. Leave for 15 minutes.

Meanwhile, put the tomatoes, onion, garlic, herbs and broth into the slow cooker, season and combine well. Set to High while you prepare the rest of the dish.

Place the spinach in a colander and run under hot water until it starts to wilt. Drain well, pressing spinach with a spoon to remove all the excess water. Tip the wilted spinach into a bowl, add the mascarpone and nutmeg, season well and mix until combined.

Place a generous spoonful of the spinach mixture onto the edge of one of the aubergine slices and roll up very carefully. Place this into the slow cooker, seam side down to hold it in place. Continue with the remaining slices.

Set the slow cooker down to Low and cook for 4–6 hours.

When you are ready to serve, remove the pot from the slow cooker. Sprinkle some Parmesan, mozzarella or mature Cheddar cheese over the rolls and place under a hot grill until the cheese is golden (skip this step if you don't eat dairy).

Serve with a lovely green salad.

This is a lovely, creamy, medium-heat curry that is delicious with cauliflower rice, although I love to serve this with lots of different dishes as part of a bigger Indian meal. If you are vegan, you can swap the paneer for tofu (both are curds: paneer is made with cow's milk; tofu is made from soybeans).

Palak Paneer

Serves 4–8

❄ 🍲 Ⓥ ⊘ ✎

Nutritional information per serving (based on serving 4)
736 Kcals
57g fat
10g net carbohydrates
43g protein

Ingredients
1 tsp coconut oil

1 small onion, finely chopped

3 garlic cloves, crushed

1 heaped tbsp grated fresh ginger

1 chilli, deseeded and finely chopped (leave seeds in if you like heat)

2 tsp ground turmeric

1 tsp mustard seeds, ground

2 tsp cardamom pods, bashed

2 tsp ground coriander

2 tsp ground cumin

½ tsp grated nutmeg

1 tsp ground cinnamon

¼ tsp cayenne pepper

300g baby leaf spinach

1 tbsp tomato purée

400ml full-fat coconut milk

200ml water or vegetable broth (if needed)

600g paneer, cut into thick chunks (use firm tofu if vegan or dairy-free)

Preheat your slow cooker, following the manufacturer's instructions.

Heat the coconut oil in a sauté pan (or use the sauté function if your slow cooker has one). Add the onion, garlic, ginger, chilli and the spices and cook over a medium heat for 3–4 minutes until the onion has softened and the spices are fragrant.

Tip the spinach into a colander and run under a hot tap to start to wilt the leaves.

Put the tomato purée, coconut milk and spinach into a food processor and whizz to create a smooth, dark green sauce. You may have to do this in batches. You can add up to 200ml water or broth if needed to help break down the spinach.

Transfer the onion and spices to the slow cooker along with the spinach and coconut milk mixture and combine well.

Add the paneer cubes, set to High and cook for 1–2 hours.

Serve as a side dish (it will feed up to 8 people) or as a main with some cauliflower rice and keto flatbreads.

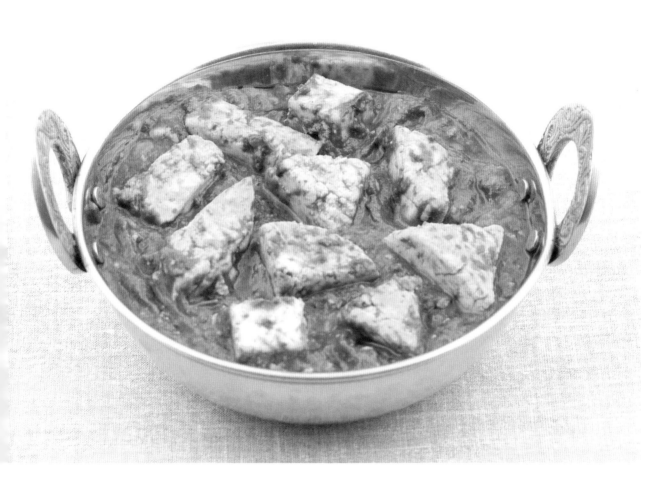

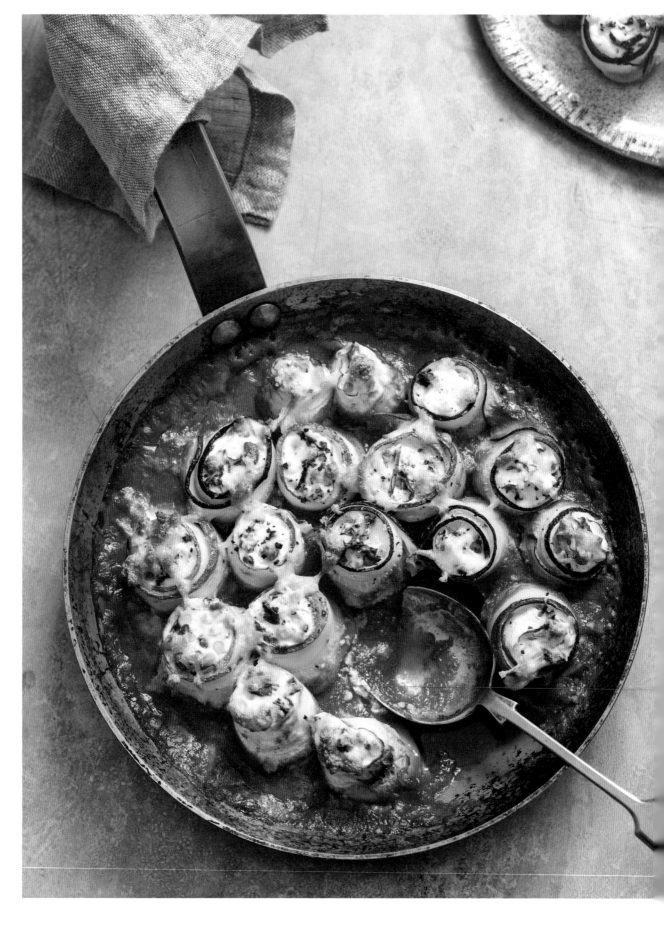

I was a vegetarian for twenty-five years and one of my favourite recipes was spinach and ricotta lasagne. Being keto means you can't eat pasta, but courgette is a wonderful option. This recipe uses thinly sliced courgette, rolled up with a spinach and ricotta mix and cooked in a rich tomato sauce in the slow cooker. It is delicious.

Spinach and Ricotta Roll-ups

Serves 4

Nutritional information per serving
441 Kcals
30g fat
11g net carbohydrates
28g protein

Ingredients
4–5 fresh tomatoes, chopped (or use 400g tin chopped tomatoes)

2 tbsp sun-dried tomato purée

1 onion, very finely chopped

2 garlic cloves, crushed

1 tsp dried thyme

1 tsp dried oregano

½ tsp dried rosemary

½ tsp dried basil

3 courgettes, thinly sliced lengthways

300g ricotta

100g baby leaf spinach

½ tsp grated nutmeg

salt and black pepper, to taste

50g mozzarella or Parmesan (optional)

Preheat your slow cooker, following the manufacturer's instructions.

Put the tomatoes, sun-dried tomato purée, half the onion, the garlic and herbs into the slow cooker. Set to High and cook for 1 hour while you prepare the roll-ups.

Boil a kettle. Pour some of the just-boiled water into a bowl or pan, add the courgette slices and leave for 2–3 minutes. This helps to soften them ready to roll.

Put the ricotta into a bowl and mash slightly with the remaining onion.

Tip the spinach into a colander or sieve and run under the hot tap until it starts to wilt slightly. Squeeze out any excess moisture using the back of a spoon, then add to the ricotta with the nutmeg and salt and to taste.

Put the courgette slices flat on the work surface. Put 2–3 teaspoons of the spinach and ricotta mixture at one end of each slice and carefully roll up; continue with all the mixture and courgette slices.

Put the rolls into the slow cooker; you can either put them in seam down into the tomato sauce or you can stand them up, as long as they are placed close together, so they do not unravel.

Turn the slow cooker down to Low and cook for another 3 hours.

If you want a nice cheesy crust on top, transfer to your ovenproof serving dish, sprinkle with mozzarella or Parmesan before placing the pan under a hot grill until the cheese is bubbling and golden.

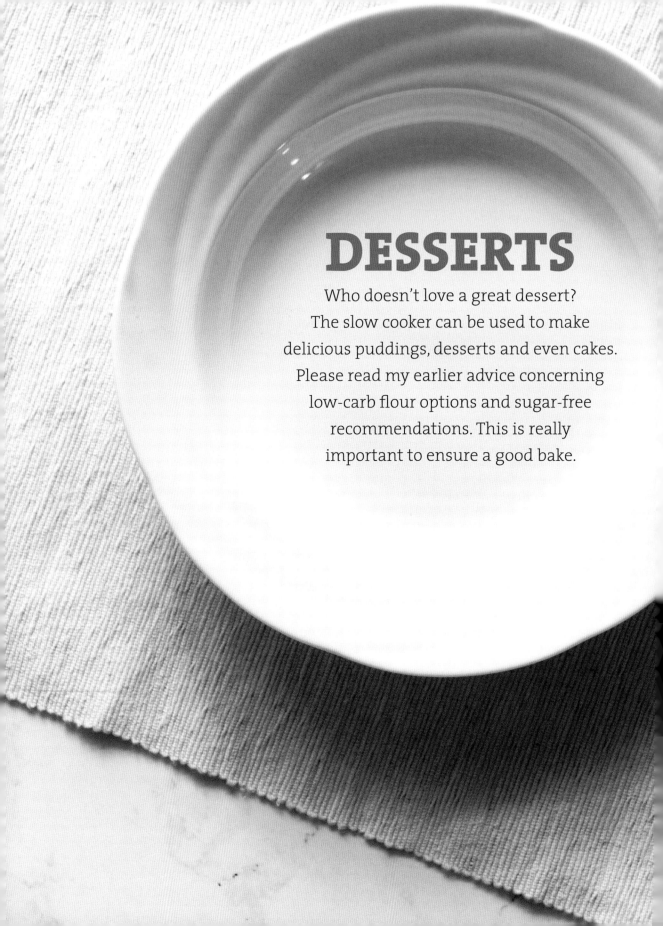

DESSERTS

Who doesn't love a great dessert?
The slow cooker can be used to make
delicious puddings, desserts and even cakes.
Please read my earlier advice concerning
low-carb flour options and sugar-free
recommendations. This is really
important to ensure a good bake.

REDUCE YOUR SUGAR INTAKE

I have worked with a number of schools where sugar intake in cakes and desserts has been reduced by 40 per cent without anyone noticing any changes. You really don't need things to be as sweet as you might think, and that also applies when you are using keto sweeteners. Start gradually and reduce, allowing you and your family to get used to fewer sweet foods, therefore reducing sweet cravings. For more information on sweeteners see the Keto Store Cupboard chapter on page 16.

FLOURS

Keto flours are mainly flours from ground nuts. You can grind your own nuts to make nut flour, which is by far the healthiest option (I use a Nutribullet to do this). Store home-ground nut flours in the freezer to prevent them going rancid.

I use coconut flour, ground almonds and a variety of other nut flours such as hazelnut. I also use flaxseeds a lot. When baking with these flours, you will need to add baking powder to make them rise. I sometimes use ground almond flour on its own but I also find combining flours works well: 3 parts hazelnut flour and 2 parts ground almonds work really well in cakes. Some people find a combination of 3 parts coconut flour and 1 part almond flour to be the best combination. If using coconut flour, you'll need to adjust the liquid as coconut flour absorbs almost ten times its volume, so if you are not careful you could have a very, very dry cake! I have found I have best results when baking with coconut flour if I use 1 egg and 2 tablespoons of liquid (milk, water, buttermilk or Greek yoghurt) per 30g coconut flour. You will also need to use less coconut flour in recipes, roughly half. It does take some getting used to. Always sift coconut flour before using as it can really clump up in the packaging.

This is an easy chocolate cake that works well in the slow cooker. It is quite rich but still maintains a lightness despite being slow-cooked. I prefer it warm served with some cream, but it is also delicious cold and is a perfect sweet treat for keto packed lunches. The thickness of the cake depends on the size of your slow cooker. I use my Ninja Foodi for this; it has a 24cm diameter pot.

Keto Rich Chocolate Cake

Makes 10 slices

Nutritional information per slice
379 Kcals
34g fat
2.9g net carbohydrates
12g protein

Ingredients
200g soft butter, plus extra for greasing

4 eggs

100g erythritol (or use monk fruit granules or stevia)

250g ground almonds

50g coconut flour

1 tsp gluten-free baking powder

60g unsweetened cocoa or cacao powder

75ml buttermilk

Preheat your slow cooker, following the manufacturer's instructions.

Grease the slow cooker pan thoroughly; alternatively, you can line it with a cake liner, slow cooker liner or baking parchment.

Put all the ingredients into a large bowl and beat well until you have a smooth cake batter. Pour this into the slow cooker and level the surface.

Set to High and cook for 2–3 hours, or until a knife placed into the centre of the cake comes out clean.

Remove the slow cooker insert from the slow cooker to allow the cake to cool for 10–15 minutes. If you have lined the slow cooker, you can just lift the cake out; if not, you need to carefully invert your serving dish over the top of the slow cooker bowl. Using oven gloves, hold both the bowl and the serving dish and flip over. The cake should drop on to the serving dish.

Serve hot or cold with a dollop of cream.

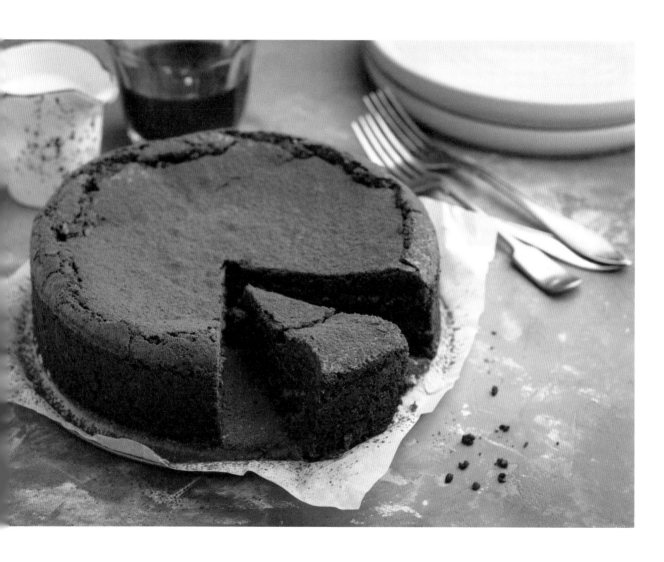

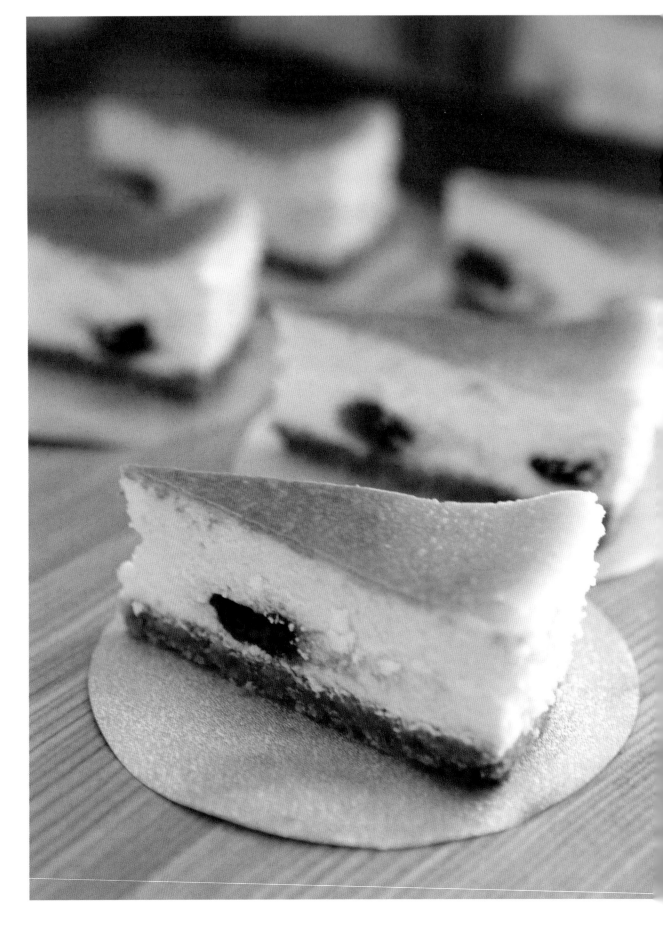

I love baked cheesecakes, and this is no exception. I have used blueberries in this recipe as they work so well with the zesty lemon, but it works really well with raspberries or just opt for plain vanilla and cut down on the lemon.

New York-style Blueberry and Lemon Cheesecake

Serves 10

Nutritional information per serving
494 Kcals
47g fat
4.3g net carbohydrates
11g protein

Ingredients
150g milled nut and seed mix (I use Yum & Yay)

40g butter, melted

2 tbsp Sukrin Fibre Syrup (optional)

4 eggs, beaten

700g full-fat cream cheese

350ml extra-thick cream

grated zest of 3 lemons

2 tsp vanilla extract

100g fresh blueberries

Preheat your slow cooker, following the manufacturer's instructions.

I use a milled nut and seed mix but you can mill nuts and seeds yourself by pulsing 100g nuts and 50g seeds in a high-speed food processor until they are of a crumby consistency. Place the milled nuts in a bowl and add the melted butter and fibre syrup (if using). Combine well.

Line the slow cooker with a cake liner, slow cooker liner or baking parchment. Tip the nut mixture into the base and spread evenly. Push down to form a solid base.

Put the remaining ingredients, apart from the blueberries, into a bowl and mix together until well combined.

Spread a little of the cream mixture on to the nut base. Add the blueberries and follow with the remaining cream mixture. Smooth the top.

Set to Low and cook for 2½–3 hours, until the top feels just firm to the touch. Leave to cool in the slow cooker before attempting to remove it.

Chill before serving.

I love comfort food, and this really hits the spot. I pick blackberries in late summer and freeze them ready to make dishes like this. You don't need many blackberries to create a fabulous flavour and bold colour, although you could substitute the blackberries for raspberries.

Blackberry Custard Pot

Serves 6

Nutritional information per serving
374 Kcals
37g fat
2.9g net carbohydrates
7.4g protein

Ingredients
4 eggs, beaten

75g erythritol (or use monk fruit granules or stevia)

grated zest of 1 lemon

200g cream cheese

300ml extra-thick cream

75g blackberries, plus a few extra to decorate

Preheat your slow cooker, following the manufacturer's instructions.

Mix the eggs, erythritol, lemon zest, cream cheese and cream together until the mixture is smooth.

Crush the blackberries and add to the egg mixture. Combine well.

Divide evenly between 6 ramekins and pop into your slow cooker. Carefully pour water from a just-boiled kettle into the slow cooker so that the water comes halfway up the sides of the ramekin dishes.

Set to Low and cook for 2–2½ hours until they are set.

Decorate each ramekin with a few whole blackberries before serving with a dollop of extra-thick cream.

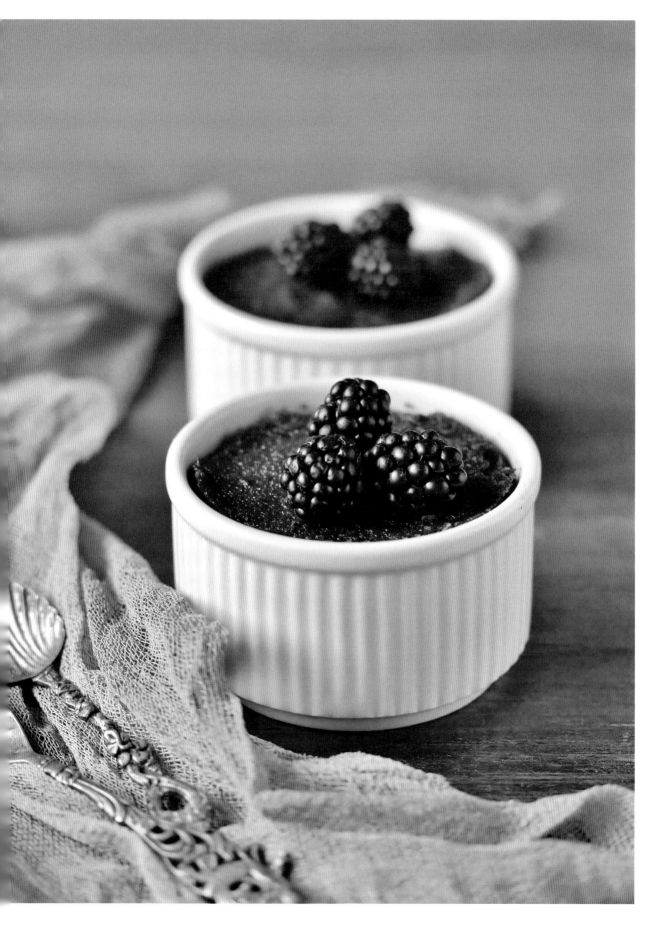

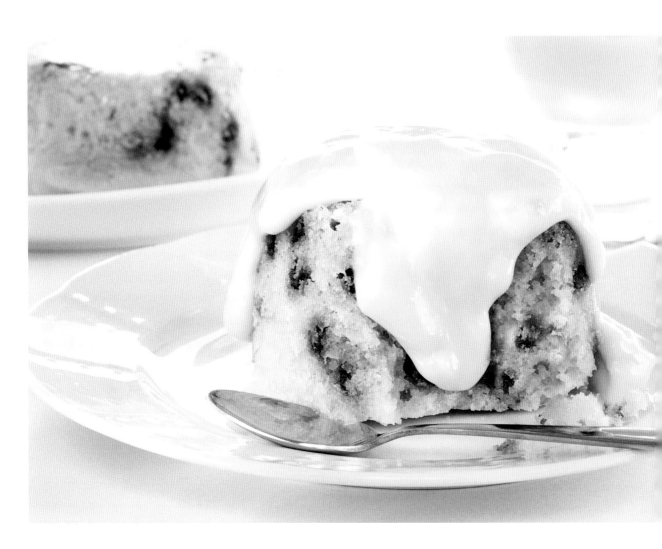

Spotted dick is a traditional sponge made with currants. It is a real classic adored by families in the UK. This is my version – ditching the currants and replacing them with sugar-free chocolate chips. You can make this in one large pudding basin (I use a 1.2 litre basin).

Keto Spotted Sponge Pudding

Serves 8

Nutritional information per serving
533 Kcals
49g fat
3.7g net carbohydrates
16g protein

You will need
1.2 litre pudding basin, baking parchment, foil and kitchen string

Ingredients
200g soft butter, plus extra for greasing

4 eggs

80g erythritol (or use monk fruit granules or stevia)

300g ground almonds

50g coconut flour

1 tsp baking powder

50ml buttermilk

75g sugar-free dark chocolate chips/drops

Preheat your slow cooker, following the manufacturer's instructions.

Grease the pudding basin generously and thoroughly with butter; this will make removing the sponge from the bowl easier.

Put all the ingredients, apart from the chocolate chips, into a large bowl. Beat well until you have a smooth cake batter. Stir in the chocolate chips.

Pour the mixture into the greased pudding basin. Cover the top with a sheet of baking parchment and then a sheet of foil and secure with string.

Place a trivet into the base of your slow cooker and put the pudding basin on top. Pour in water from a just-boiled kettle until it reaches halfway up the side of the pudding basin.

Set to High and cook for 1 hour, then check. The pudding should have a golden sponge topping which is firm to touch.

Serve immediately with keto custard or a dollop of extra-thick cream,

So simple but totally delicious and a perfect dessert for a dinner party. These can be made in advance and stored in the fridge until you are ready to caramelise the top and serve. If you are dairy-free, you can make these with coconut cream.

Lemon and Raspberry Crème Brûlée

Serves 6

Nutritional information per serving
383 Kcals
40g fat
1.8g net carbohydrates
3.3g protein

You will need
6 ramekin dishes

Ingredients
400ml double cream (or use coconut cream if dairy-free)

4 egg yolks

1 tsp vanilla extract

grated zest of 3 lemons

40g Sukrin Gold (erythritol), plus 4 tsp for the topping (or use xylitol blend)

100g raspberries, plus a few extra to decorate

a few fresh mint sprigs, to decorate

Preheat your slow cooker, following the manufacturer's recommendations.

Put the cream and egg yolks into a bowl and whisk to combine – I use a hand-held electric whisk for this. Add the vanilla extract, lemon zest and sweetener and combine again.

Divide the raspberries evenly between six ramekin dishes and then pour the creamy mixture into each of the ramekin dishes.

Place the ramekin dishes in the slow cooker and carefully pour water from a just-boiled kettle around the edges of the ramekin dishes so that the water comes about halfway up the sides of the ramekins.

Set to Low and bake for 2–3 hours, or until they start to set – they won't be totally firm. Remove from the slow cooker and set aside to cool. I normally leave these in the fridge for at least 1 hour before serving.

When you are ready to serve, sprinkle the top of each ramekin with a little erythritol, then use a kitchen blowtorch to caramelise the top, taking care not to burn them.

Decorate each ramekin with some raspberries and a sprig of fresh mint.

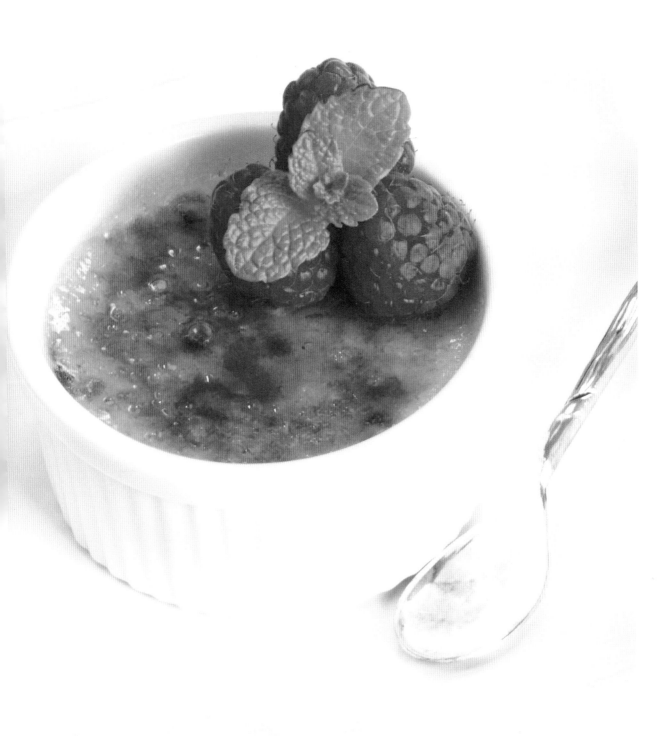

EXTRAS &
SIDE DISHES

When you are following a ketogenic way
of eating, you have to calculate or monitor
all your carbohydrates.

The slow cooker recipes in this book all include nutritional analysis but what about the meal accompaniments? This way of eating means no more potatoes, pasta, rice or bread so it can be quite hard to visualise your favourite family meals done the keto way.

You can, of course, just go for steamed green vegetables and salads but I hope this chapter will inspire you to make the most of your slow cooker meals as it includes my favourite keto side dishes

Cauliflower is so versatile. It is a real staple for the ketogenic way of eating. We hear so much about cauliflower rice, but people are often confused about how to cook it correctly. I use cauliflower rice a lot, but also broccoli rice, which has a milder, more nutty flavour. The consistency is similar to couscous and there are a few ways to cook this: in the microwave, sautéed or steamed; you can also roast whole florets on a baking tray before zapping in a food processor. I usually use either the sauté or microwave options as they are really easy. If you prefer the flavour of broccoli, just cook in the same way.

Cauliflower Rice

Serves 4

Nutritional
information per
serving
39 Kcals
0.4g fat
4.8g net carbohydrates
2g fibre
2.8g protein

Ingredients
1 whole cauliflower

Trim off the leaves and stalks from the cauliflower, and cut or break the cauliflower into florets.

Put the florets into a food processor and pulse for a few minutes until the cauliflower resembles rice. If you don't have a processor you can grate this using the large holes of a box grater, but it is messy and more time-consuming.

TO COOK IN THE MICROWAVE

When you are ready to cook, put the cauliflower rice into a lidded container, without any water, and pop into the microwave.

Cook on full power for 5–8 minutes (cooking times will depend on your microwave). Stir halfway through cooking to ensure an even cook.

Remove and fluff up with a fork; serve immediately.

TO SAUTÉ ON THE HOB

Heat a little butter or coconut oil in sauté pan.

Add the cauliflower rice and toss gently over a medium heat for 5–8 minutes until heated through and softened.

Serve immediately.

Top Tip
Whizz up a few cauliflowers at a time and place the uncooked, processed cauliflower rice into freezer bags. You can then cook this from frozen, using which-ever method you prefer.

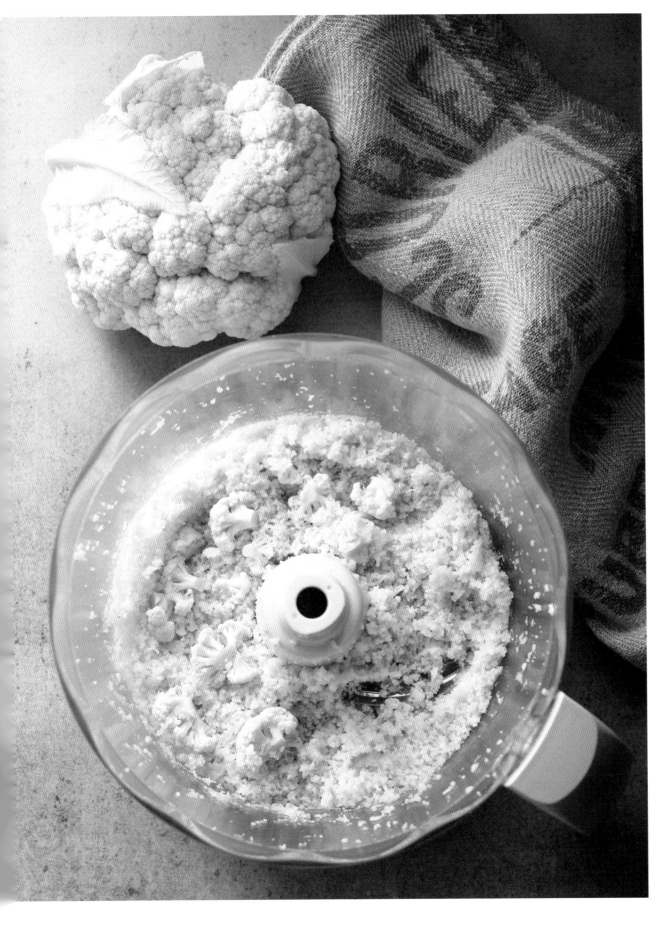

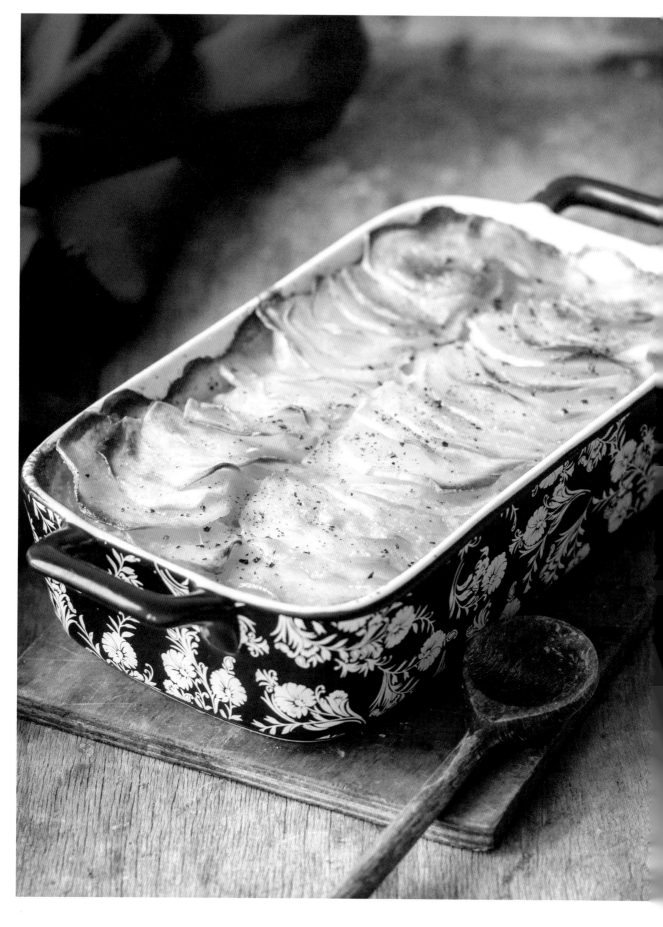

Just like cauliflower, celeriac is a great addition to the keto way of eating. The secret to success with this side dish is to slice your celeriac as thinly as possible, ideally using a food processor or mandoline. I make this a lot for dinner parties as I can prep it in advance and bake when ready. It is a brilliant accompaniment to beef bourguignon or a roast dinner.

Celeriac Dauphinoise

Serves 6

Nutritional information per serving
535 Kcals
53g fat
3.3g net carbohydrates
9g protein

Ingredients
1 large celeriac (about 400g), peeled

4 garlic cloves, crushed

500ml double cream (or use coconut cream if dairy-free)

½ tsp grated nutmeg

salt and black pepper, to taste

150g Gruyère cheese, grated (omit if dairy-free)

Using a food processor or mandoline, slice the celeriac as thinly as possible, ideally 1–2mm thick. Transfer the slices to a large saucepan.

Add the garlic, cream and nutmeg and season with black pepper to taste.

Place over a medium heat and allow the cream to heat up. Watch this as you don't want it to burn or stick. You will have more celeriac than liquid, so it is important that you move the celeriac occasionally to ensure a more even cook. Simmer gently for 5 minutes.

Remove the pan from the heat and carefully transfer the celeriac slices to an ovenproof dish. Top with the cream mixture.

Finish with the grated Gruyère and season with salt and pepper. You can keep this in the fridge until needed. When you are ready to cook, preheat the oven to 170°C (150°C fan) Gas 3. I find it easier to place the ovenproof dish on to a baking tray (just in case it spills over during cooking); you can then slide this on to the middle shelf of the oven. Cook for 30–40 minutes until golden.

I love roast dinners and roast potatoes were a big favourite of mine before I started following the keto way of eating. However, I can honestly say I no longer miss them thanks to celeriac roast potatoes. I cook them in the same way as roast potatoes, and they are absolutely delicious. Serve with your roasted or slow-cooked joint and steamed vegetables.

Celeriac Roast Potatoes

Serves 4

Nutritional information per serving
109 Kcals
11g fat
0.9g net carbohydrates
0.5g protein

Ingredients
1 celeriac (about 300g), peeled

2–3 tbsp goose fat

1 tsp paprika

2–3 sprigs of thyme

2 garlic cloves, peeled but left whole

sea salt

Preheat the oven to 190°C (170°C) Gas 5 and bring a large saucepan of water to the boil.

Peel the celeriac before cutting into large potato-sized chunks. Add to the pan of boiling water and cook for 10 minutes.

Meanwhile, put the goose fat into a roasting tray and pop into the oven to heat up.

Drain the celeriac. Remove the roasting tray from the oven and carefully put the drained celeriac into the hot fat. Sprinkle with paprika then add the thyme and garlic.

Roast for 1–1½ hours until golden and crisp. Transfer to a serving dish and sprinkle with sea salt before serving.

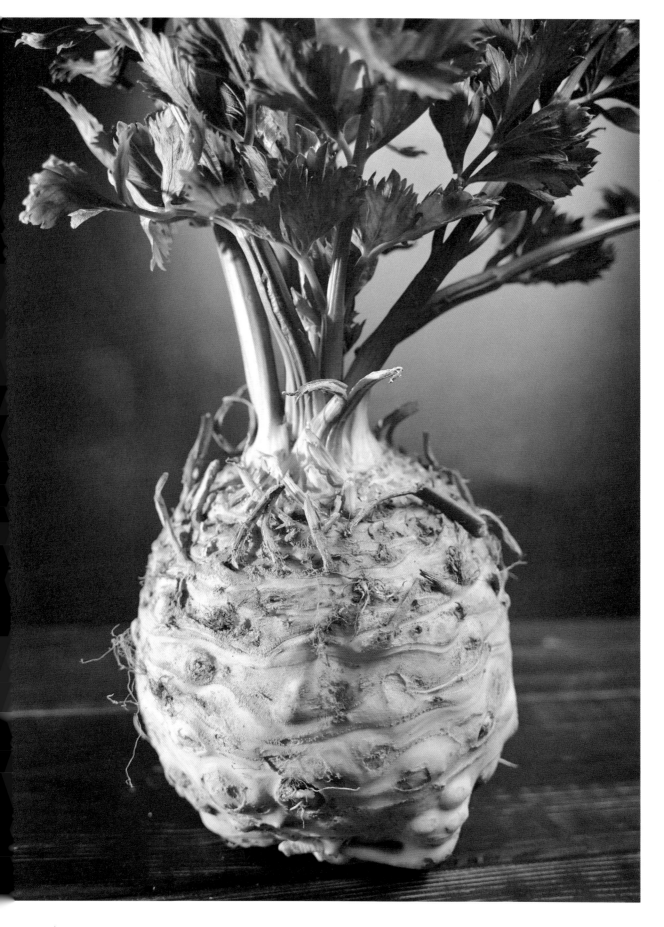

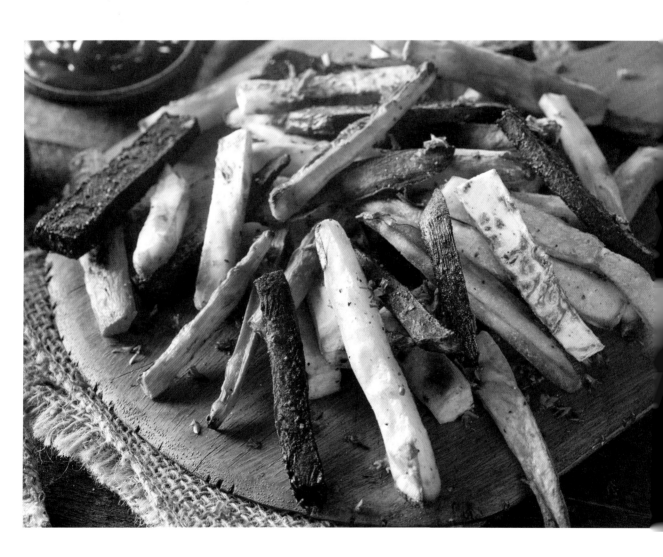

You can make keto fries using swede, celeriac or even haloumi. They work best when you use an air fryer (a kitchen appliance that works by circulating hot air around the food) but if you don't have one, you could cook these in the oven with a little coconut or goose fat for 30–40 minutes until crispy.

Keto Fries

To make fries using swede or celeriac, you need to cut the vegetable into thick 'chips'. Soak them in cold water for at least 10 minutes before patting dry with kitchen towel.

If using halloumi, pat dry with kitchen towel before cutting into thick chips.

When you are ready to cook, place your chips in the air fryer and cook on High. Halloumi fries will take about 15–20 minutes; vegetables such as celeriac or swede take up to 30 minutes to cook, depending on the thickness of the chips.

I love my cauliflower mash with lots of butter and mature cheese. It is a very simple recipe, taking minutes when cooked in the microwave and ideal as a meal accompaniment, but also as a topping to your cottage pie or fish pie. If you prefer not to use a microwave, you can roast or steam the cauliflower first before mashing. And you can also use the same method to make celeriac or swede mash – or a mixture of both!

Cauliflower Mash

Serves 4

Nutritional information per serving
140 Kcals
11g fat
4.4g net carbohydrates
6.2g protein

Ingredients
1 whole cauliflower (about 250g)
20g butter
75g mature Cheddar, grated
salt and black pepper, to taste

Trim off the leaves and stalks from the cauliflower, then break or cut into florets.

Place the florets into a food processor and pulse for a few minutes until the cauliflower resembles rice. If you don't have a food processor you can grate this using the large holes of a box grater, but it is messy and more time-consuming.

When you are ready to cook, place the cauliflower rice in a lidded container, without any water, and pop into the microwave.

Cook on full power for 5–8 minutes, depending on your microwave's heat settings. Stir halfway through cooking to ensure an even cook.

Remove and mash up with a fork. Add the butter and cheese and continue to mash with your fork until it is all combined. Season to taste and serve immediately.

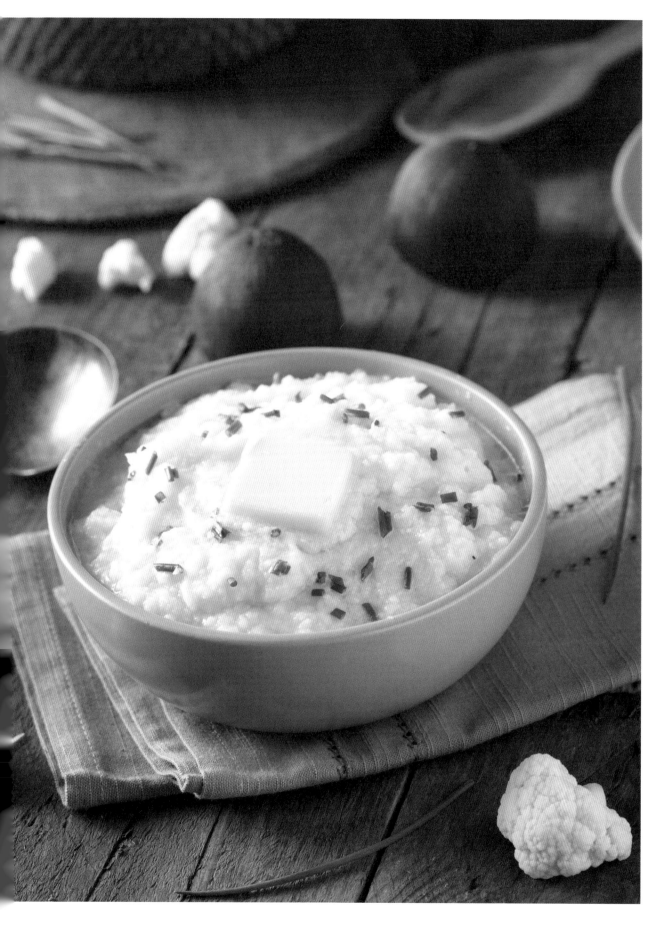

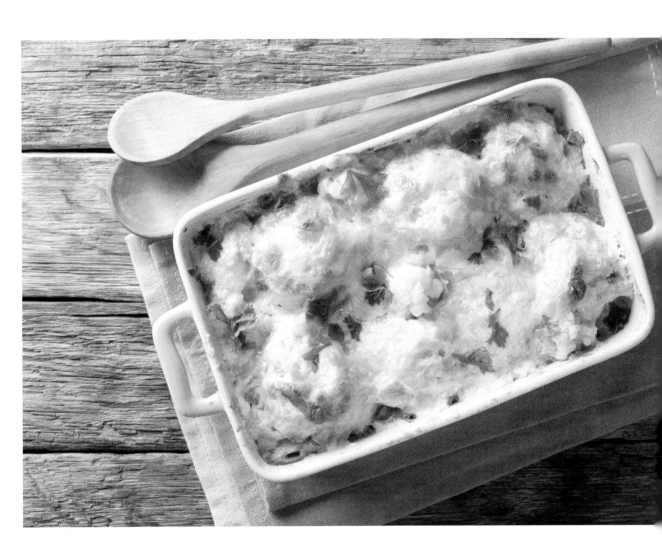

Cauliflower cheese is one of my favourites; I eat this a lot. The cheese sauce takes minutes to make and is so simple. You can use this sauce recipe for a variety of meals so it's useful to have in your keto repertoire.

Cauliflower Cheese

Serves 4

Nutritional information per serving
292 Kcals
25g fat
6.6g net carbohydrates
10g protein

Ingredients
1 cauliflower (about 250g)

300g cream cheese

100ml full-fat milk or double cream

75–100g mature Cheddar, grated, plus extra for topping

salt and black pepper, to taste

Cut your cauliflower into florets and steam them until they are only just soft.

Put the cream cheese into a saucepan with the milk or cream and heat gently. Once heated, add the grated cheese and season with black pepper. Stir over a medium-low heat until the cheese is melted. Be careful not to heat up too much or it will stick and burn.

Once the cheese is melted, taste and adjust by adding more cheese or seasoning to suit.

Tip the steamed cauliflower into an ovenproof dish and pour over the cheese sauce. You can eat this now or, if you prefer, you can add some grated cheese and place under a hot grill until golden and bubbling.

Top Tip
Use this cheese sauce recipe to make leeks in cheese sauce, or leeks wrapped in bacon. I also use it in my lasagna, or it is delicious served with some thick gammon slices.

You will be surprised how easy these wraps are to make. They can be made in advance and, if stored in an airtight container between sheets of kitchen towel, retain their softness for 48 hours. They are great for chicken fajitas, but also good for packed lunches – my favourite is salad, chicken, avocado and bacon. These wraps are plain but if you want something with a bit of flavour, you can add some spices or flavourings to taste, such as dried herbs, onion powder, paprika or turmeric.

Keto Wraps

Serves 4

Nutritional information per serving
567 Kcals
46g fat
1.5g net carbohydrates
22g protein

Ingredients
400g milled flaxseeds or milled seeds
salt and black pepper or spices, to taste
150–200ml boiling water
coconut flour, for dusting

Put the milled flaxseeds into a bowl. Add salt and pepper or your chosen flavourings to taste.

Boil your kettle. Add a little of the just-boiled water at a time to the bowl until the flaxseeds start to form a dough. Leave to sit for 10 minutes.

When it has cooled, cut the dough into 4 equal pieces. Place one piece at a time in the centre of a sheet of baking parchment lightly dusted with coconut flour.

Place another piece of baking parchment over the top and roll out into a circle – you are aiming for the same size and thickness of traditional wraps (15–20cm in diameter). Be careful not to go too thin as the dough is quite delicate so can break easily. I like to leave the wrap on the parchment until I am ready to cook. Repeat with the other pieces of dough.

When you are ready to cook, place a large frying pan, ideally slightly larger than your wrap, over a medium heat. Add a little coconut oil and once melted, flip your wrap on to the frying pan – you can then very gently peel off the parchment. Cook on both sides for 1–2 minutes until they start to go slightly golden.

Transfer to kitchen towel and leave to cool. Store in an airtight container with kitchen towel between each wrap until ready to use.

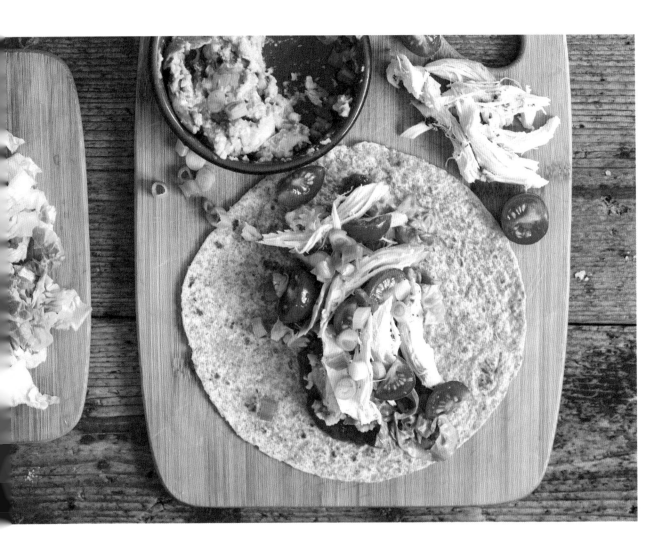

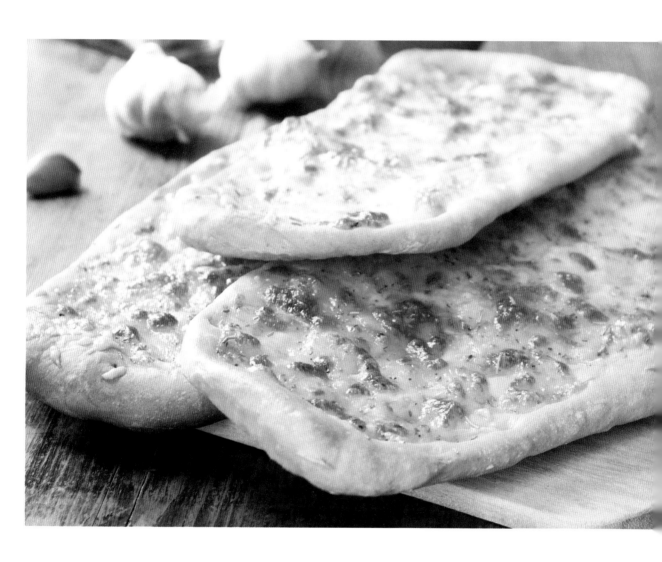

This recipe uses my special dough recipe. It's so versatile; I make pizza bases, cinnamon rolls and my favourite savoury pinwheels using this dough. Cheesy garlic bread is one of my son's favourites – he loves it with courgetti bolognaise.

Cheesy Garlic Bread

Makes 4 breads (serving 8)

Nutritional information per pizza base
434 Kcals
38g fat
1.8g net carbohydrates
20g protein

You will need
2–3 large baking sheets, baking parchment

Ingredients
250g Cheddar, grated (or use mozzarella)

100g full-fat cream cheese

2 eggs

220g ground almonds

½ tsp garlic powder

1 tsp dried oregano

salt and black pepper, to taste

50g butter, softened

3 garlic cloves, crushed

100g grated mozzarella

Preheat the oven to 170°C (150°C) Gas 3.

Put the grated Cheddar and cream cheese into a bowl and pop into the microwave for 1 minute to soften (this makes it easier to form into a dough).

Remove from the microwave and add the eggs, ground almonds, garlic powder, oregano and salt and pepper and mix well to combine. This will form a wet dough – similar to a wet scone mix.

Form into a ball and cut into 4 pieces – one for each flat garlic bread.

Place a large sheet of baking parchment on the worktop, add a ball of dough to the centre of the parchment and place another sheet of parchment on top of the dough. Press down with your hands to gently flatten – this is the easiest way to form the base without getting sticky hands and worktop! Press into a flatbread shape using your hands and knuckles. The dough needs to be about 1cm thick.

Place the whole thing, including parchment, on to a baking sheet before removing the top sheet of parchment. Repeat with the remaining dough portions.

Mix the butter and garlic together and spread this over the dough circles. Finish with the grated mozzarella.

Pop into the oven and cook for 15–20 minutes until the tops start to go golden. Serve immediately.

PANTRY ESSENTIALS

The slow cooker is so versatile – it is not just for casseroles and soups! This chapter includes some vital keto essentials that can be cooked in bulk and stored in your fridge, freezer or pantry until needed.

The keto way of eating means avoiding food with added sugar. Unfortunately many spice blends, pastes and sauces contain added sugar so we have to make our own. Here are my favourites, which help to transform your family favourite meals to keto with ease.

This is a really healthy broth; much better for you than using processed stock cubes. It is packed with minerals such as calcium, magnesium and phosphorus, as well as collagen, glucosamine and hyaluronic acid and a wide range of vitamins. It helps support the digestive tract, boosts the immune system, reduces inflammation, strengthens joints, hair and nails and promotes healthy skin. Speak to your butcher as they are often happy to give away bones for you to use.

Bone Broth

Makes 2–3 litres, depending on what you use

Ingredients
1kg bones (e.g. bone marrow, ribs, knuckles)

100ml apple cider vinegar

2 large onions, quartered

2 garlic cloves, roughly chopped

2 carrots, roughly chopped (optional)

2–3 celery sticks, roughly chopped

2 tsp mixed herbs

a small handful of fresh parsley (or 2–3 tsp dried)

2–3 bay leaves

2 tsp black peppercorns

If you are using meaty bones, you can roast them first to help release the flavours and nutrients, although this step isn't absolutely necessary. Preheat the oven to 180°C (160°C fan) Gas 4, then roast the bones for 45 minutes.

Preheat your slow cooker, following the manufacturer's instructions.

Put all the ingredients into your slow cooker and cover with water.

Set to Low and cook for 24 hours (for bones that have been roasted) or up to 48 hours for raw bones.

You may want to occasionally remove any scum from the surface of the water (this is perfectly normal). I use a slotted spoon and just scoop it out.

When cooked, remove the insert from the slow cooker and carefully strain the broth. Leave it to cool and settle; it will form a layer of fat on the top once cooled but you can just scrape this off – don't discard this as it can be used as a cooking fat.

Transfer to a container to keep in the fridge, or portion into ziplock freezer bags or silicone ice-cube trays to freeze, ready to use in your everyday dishes.

Top Tip
I store my broth in ziplock freezer bags and in large silicone ice-cube trays. The freezer bags can be defrosted quickly by popping the sealed bag into a bowl of water. I use the ice-cube trays to pop out a few small ice stock 'cubes' to add to dishes such as a chilli or spaghetti bolognese.

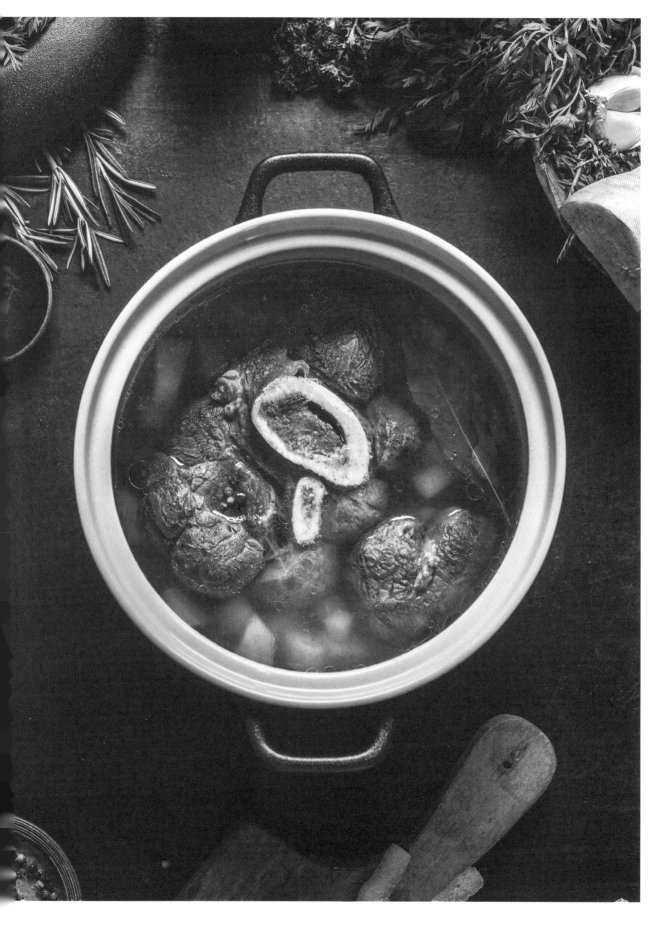

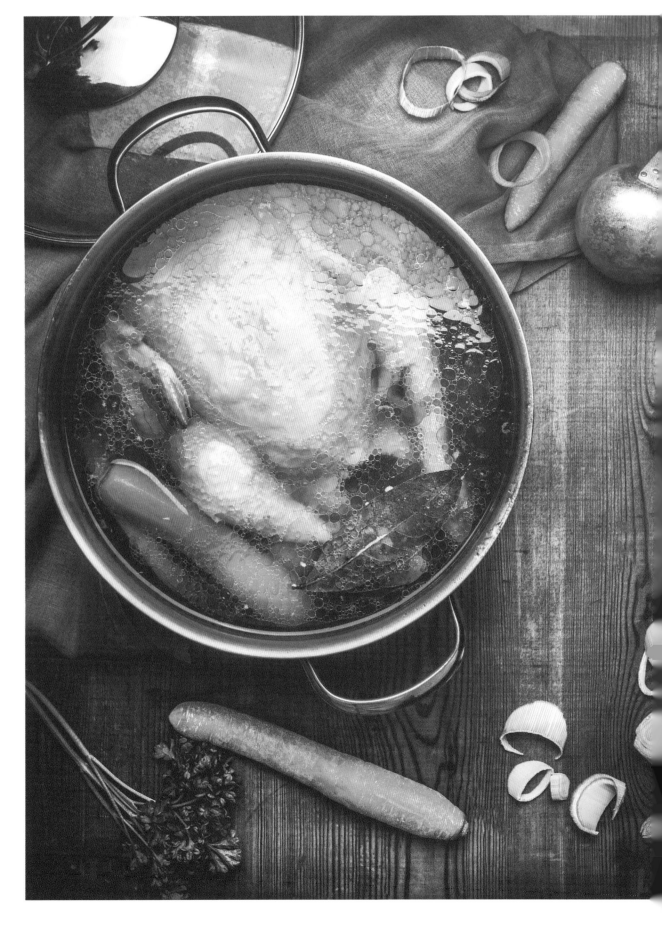

This is similar in principle to the bone broth on page 162, but chicken bones do not need as long a cook. If your chicken is already roasted, you can reduce the cooking time to 8–12 hours.

Chicken Broth

Serves 4
Ø

Ingredients
1 chicken carcass

1 large onion, quartered

1 carrot, roughly chopped

2–3 celery sticks, roughly chopped

2 tsp dried thyme

a small handful of fresh parsley (or 2–3 tsp dried)

2–3 bay leaves

2 tsp black peppercorns

Preheat your slow cooker, following the manufacturer's instructions.

Put all the ingredients into your slow cooker and cover with water.

Set to Low and cook for 12–24 hours.

When cooked, remove the insert from the slow cooker and carefully strain the broth through a sieve (you need to make sure you remove any tiny bones).

Transfer to a container to keep in the fridge, or portion into ziplock freezer bags or silicone ice-cube trays to freeze, ready to use in your everyday dishes.

I love cheese with a nice chutney. My olive tapenade works well (see page 170), but I was keen to recreate a real chutney. I had a glut of tomatoes this year so decided to try a new recipe in the slow cooker. If eaten in large quantities this is not really keto as it works out around 12g carbohydrates per 100g, but adding a small dollop to your favourite meal is a real treat and can work on a ketogenic way of eating.

Tomato and Courgette Chutney

Makes about 1.5kg

Ⓧ

Nutritional information per 15g serving
7 Kcals
0g fat
1.8g net carbohydrates
0g protein

Ingredients
2 red onions, finely chopped

4 garlic cloves, crushed

4cm piece of fresh ginger, grated

1–2 red chillies, deseeded and finely chopped

1kg tomatoes, quartered

2 courgettes, diced

1 tsp mustard seeds

4 cardamom pods

1 tsp smoked paprika

100ml apple cider vinegar

150g Sukrin Gold

salt and black pepper, to taste

Preheat your slow cooker, following the manufacturer's instructions.

Place all the ingredients into your slow cooker and combine well to ensure they are evenly distributed.

Set to Low and cook for 8–10 hours.

Meanwhile sterilise your jars – you'll probably need 3 average-sized jars. Wash them (and their lids) well in soapy water, rinse and then place in a low oven to dry out for about 20 minutes.

Allow the chutney to cool slightly and then transfer to your sterilised jars. Add the lids and store in the fridge until needed.

Once opened the chutney will last for a few weeks in the fridge (as the chutney does not contain sugar it may not last as long as conventional chutney).

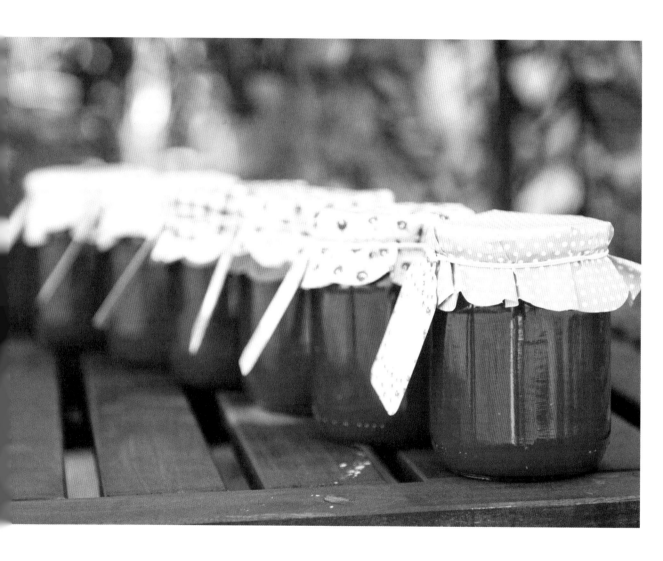

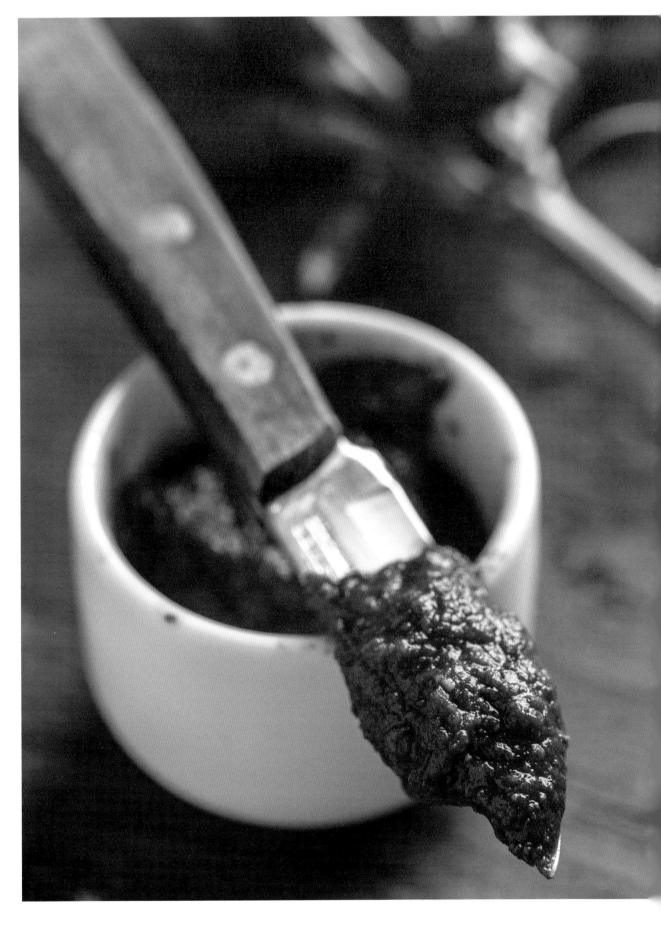

I love Moroccan flavours as they can transform a dish. I use this paste in casseroles and soups but also rub it onto my meat to create new flavours. One of my favourite dishes with this paste is a traybake, with chicken thighs coated in the paste, placed in a baking tray with Mediterranean vegetables and baked until golden. I use this a lot, so I often double or triple the quantities here. It freezes well but also keeps in the fridge, in an airtight container, for up to 4 weeks.

Spiced Harissa Paste

Dairy-free

Nutritional
information per
15g serving
21 Kcals
1.6g fat
0.9g net carbohydrates
0.5g protein

Ingredients
2 red peppers, halved
deseeded

4 tbsp olive oil, plus
extra for drizzling

2 tbsp coriander seeds

1 tbsp cumin seeds

1 tbsp fennel seeds

½ tbsp caraway seeds

6 garlic cloves

4 chillies, deseeded
(unless you like it hot!)

1 heaped tbsp smoked
paprika

1 tbsp apple cider
vinegar

2 heaped tbsp tomato
purée

Preheat the oven to 180°C (160°C fan) Gas 4.

Place the peppers on to a baking tray. Drizzle with some olive oil and pop into the oven for 20 minutes.

Meanwhile, toast the seeds in a sauté pan for 2–3 minutes. Leave to one side.

Once the peppers have been roasted put them into a food processor with all the remaining ingredients and whizz to a paste.

Transfer to a sterilised jar (see page 166) and top with a little more olive oil – this helps it stay fresher in the fridge, where it will keep for up to 4 weeks. Alternatively, you can place straight into silicone ice-cube trays and freeze, ready to pop out when needed.

A tapenade is so versatile and is great added to courgette spaghetti, on roasted vegetables or served as a dip. I love this with cheese as a keto replacement for a chutney. I have used black olives in this recipe, but you can use green if you like. I like my tapenade to have a touch of chilli heat, but you can leave out the chilli if you prefer a milder taste.

Olive Tapenade

Makes about 300g

Nutritional information per 15g serving
47 Kcals
4.4g fat
0.8g net carbohydrates
0.7g protein

Ingredients
200g pitted black Kalamata olives

2 garlic cloves, halved

1–2 red or green chillies, to taste, deseeded (optional)

1 tbsp capers

40g whole almonds

2 tbsp olive oil

1 tbsp coconut aminos

zest and juice of ½ lemon

a small handful of parsley leaves

salt and black pepper

Put all the ingredients, except the salt and pepper, into a food processor or Nutribullet and whizz until it forms a smooth paste. You may need to stop halfway through processing and scrape down the sides of the processor, then whizz again to ensure it is all well combined.

Taste and season – I love to add lots of black pepper.

Store in an airtight container, adding a little olive oil to the top to help it last. This will keep in the fridge for up to 2 weeks.

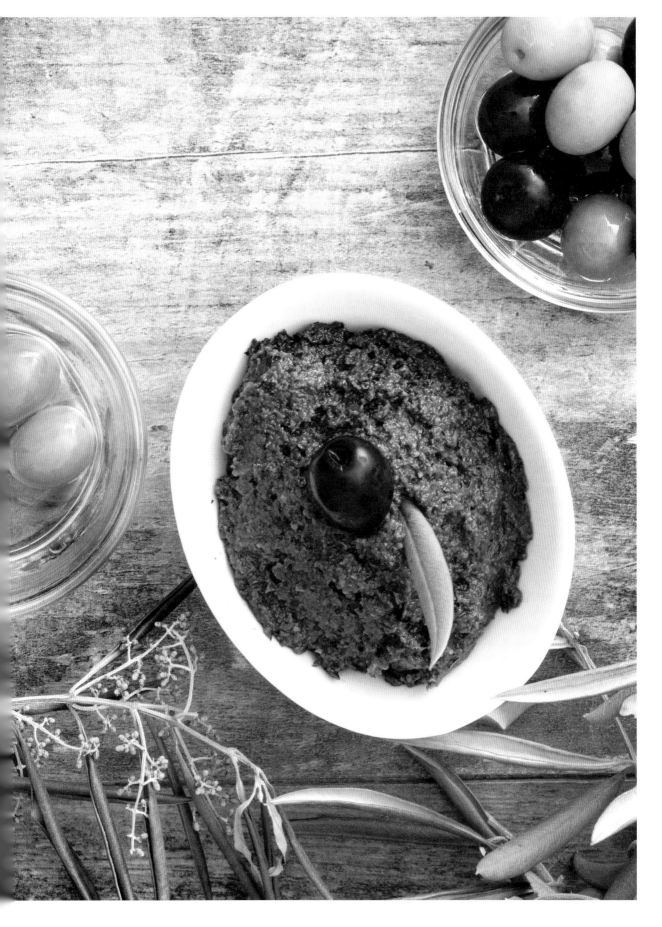

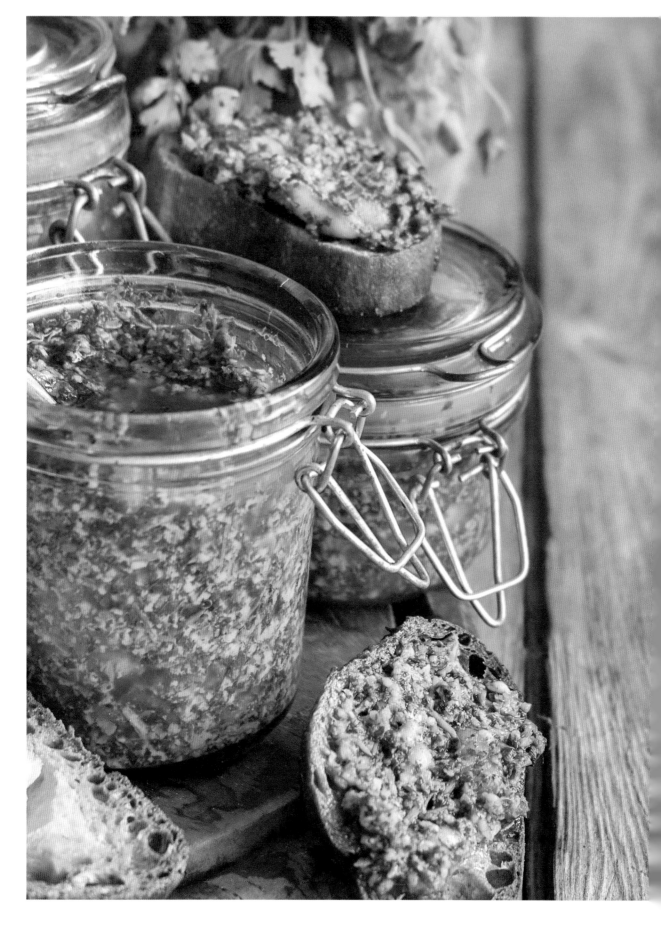

There is no reason why pesto can't have a bit of a kick and this one certainly delivers. This pesto adds a powerful zing to everyday recipes. Warning: it can be very addictive!

Chilli and Coriander Pesto

Makes about 250g

Nutritional information per 15g serving
56 Kcals
5.5g fat
0.5g net carbohydrates
1.1g protein

Ingredients
1–2 chillies

a large handful of fresh coriander

60g baby leaf spinach

75g pine nuts

3–4 garlic cloves

20g finely grated Parmesan

3–5 tbsp extra-virgin olive oil

salt and black pepper, to taste

Put all the ingredients into a food processor or blender and whizz until smooth and combined.

Pour into a dish, cover and place in the fridge for at least 30 minutes (this allows the flavours to infuse). Store in the fridge in an airtight container until ready to use. You can also freeze this – I often freeze it in silicone ice-cube trays so I can pop out a few cubes when I need them.

I love spicy food; anything with a kick is great. This is an everyday, medium curry paste – not too hot, but enough to give great flavour. You can adjust the amount of chillies depending on your taste. This is such as great paste, all you need to do is add it to your favourite meat, vegetable or fish with some coconut milk for a creamy, delicious curry.

Everyday Curry Paste

Makes about 250g
⊘

Nutritional information per 15g serving
33 Kcals
2.1g fat
1.5g net carbohydrates
0.9g protein

Ingredients
1 tbsp fennel seeds
1 tbsp mustard seeds
2 tbsp cumin seeds
4 tbsp coriander seeds
6 cardamom pods
2 tsp fenugreek seeds
1 tsp black peppercorns
1 tbsp ground turmeric
2 tsp mild chilli powder
2 tsp ground cinnamon
1 tbsp paprika
3 red chillies, deseeded
4cm piece of fresh ginger
4 curry leaves
1 tbsp tomato purée
5 garlic cloves
2 tbsp apple cider vinegar
3 tbsp olive oil, plus extra for topping
a small handful of fresh coriander

Put the seeds and peppercorns into a sauté pan and place over a medium heat for 2 minutes, until fragrant and aromatic.

Transfer to a food processor and add all the remaining ingredients, then whizz until it forms a smooth paste.

Transfer to a sterilised jar (see page 166) and add a little olive oil on top of the paste to help it last. This will keep in the fridge for up to 2 weeks. You can also freeze this – I often freeze it in silicone ice-cube trays and pop out a few cubes when I need them.

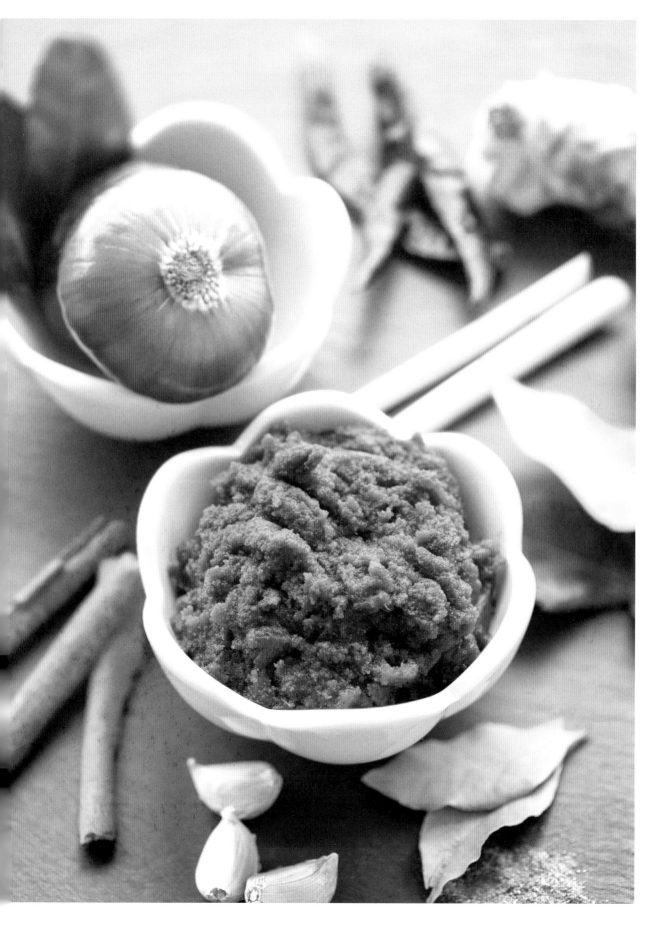

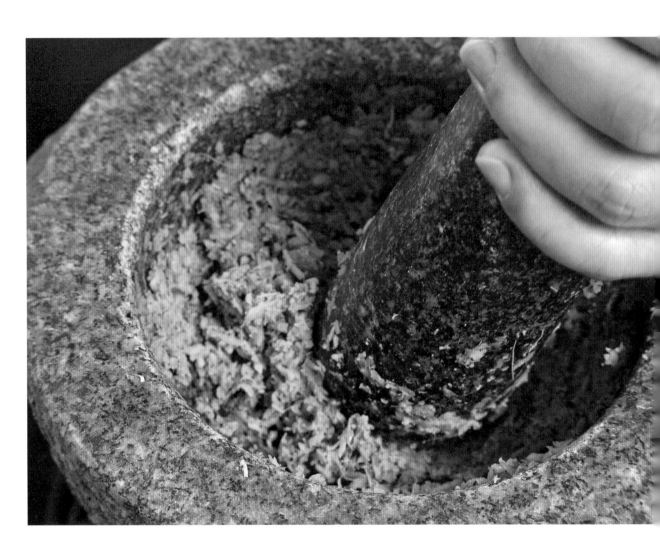

This is a lovely paste that works well with coconut milk-based curries. My son loves my Thai green curry, made using this paste, coconut milk, chicken and onion – so simple yet utterly delicious. Just like the other pastes, you can make more and freeze in ice-cube trays, ready to pop out when needed.

Thai Green Curry Paste

Makes 1 small jar

Nutritional information per 15g serving
31 Kcals
2.9g fat
0.7g net carbohydrates
0.5g protein

Ingredients
1 tbsp cumin seeds

1 tbsp coriander seeds

4 tbsp olive oil, plus extra for topping

3 green chillies, finely chopped

½ small white onion

4 garlic cloves

4cm piece of fresh ginger

2 lemongrass stalks, trimmed

3 dried kaffir lime leaves

1 tbsp fish sauce

grated zest and juice of 1 lime

a small bunch of fresh coriander

Put the seeds into a sauté pan and place over a medium heat for 2 minutes until fragrant and aromatic.

Transfer to a food processor and add all the remaining ingredients, then whizz until it forms a smooth paste.

Pop into a sterilised jar (see page 166) and add a little olive oil on top of the paste to help it last. This will keep in the fridge for up to 2 weeks. You can also freeze this – I normally freeze it in silicone ice-cube trays and pop out a few cubes when I need them.

This is a great paste that can add flavour to a lot of dishes, from chicken to soups; it's also delicious with prawns. If you don't like things too hot, you may want to adjust the chilli content and switch the hot paprika to standard paprika.

Thai Red Curry Paste

Makes 1 small jar
Ⓥ

Nutritional information per 15g serving
39 Kcals
3.6g fat
0.9g net carbohydrates
0.5g protein

Ingredients
1 tbsp cumin seeds

1 tbsp coriander seeds

4 tbsp olive oil, plus extra for topping

3 red chillies, finely chopped

4 garlic cloves

½ red onion

4cm piece of fresh ginger

2 lemongrass stalks, trimmed

grated zest and juice of 1 lime

2 tbsp hot paprika

5 sun-dried tomatoes, drained of oil

Put the seeds into a sauté pan and place over a medium heat for 2 minutes until fragrant and aromatic.

Transfer to a food processor, add all the remaining ingredients and whizz to a smooth paste.

Pop into a sterilised jar (see page 166) and add a little olive oil on top of the paste to help it last. This will keep in the fridge for up to 2 weeks. You can also freeze this – I normally freeze it in silicone ice-cube trays and pop out a few cubes when I need them.

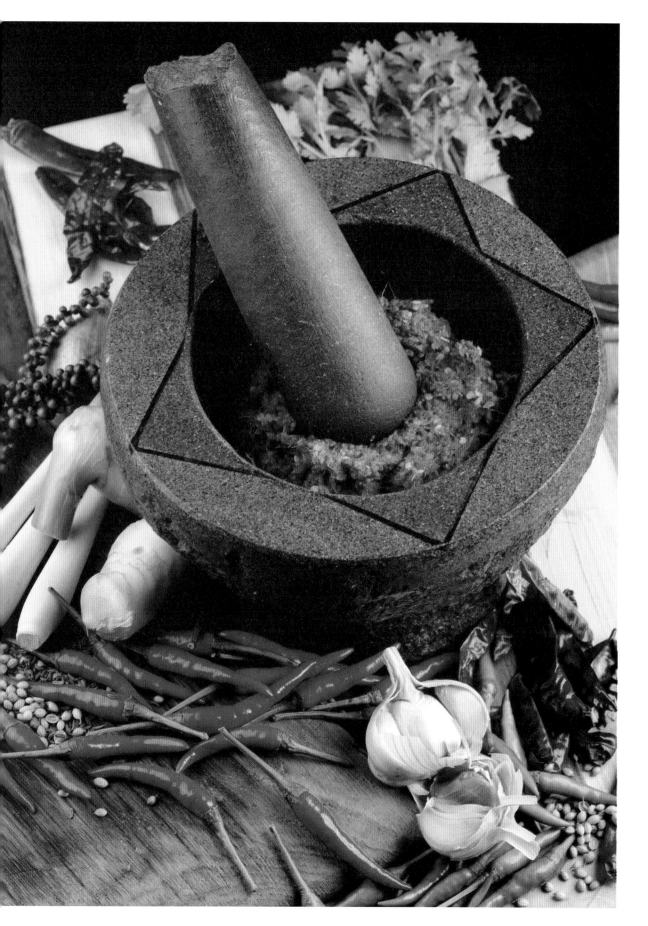

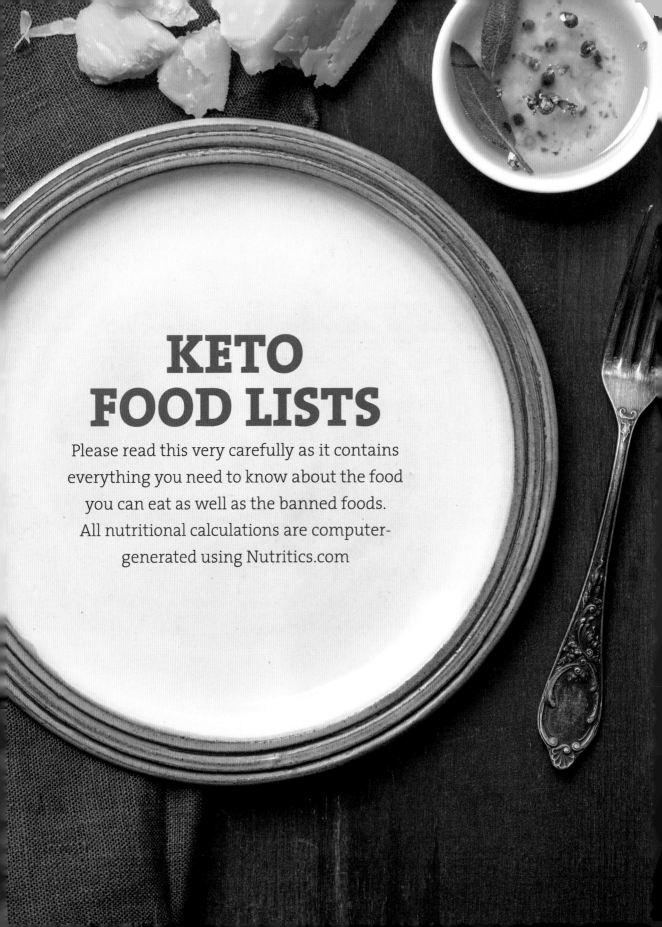

KETO
FOOD LISTS

Please read this very carefully as it contains
everything you need to know about the food
you can eat as well as the banned foods.
All nutritional calculations are computer-
generated using Nutritics.com

Staple low-carb and ketogenic foods

Just as the title implies, this list contains all the foods you can eat when following a low-carb or ketogenic way of eating. The ideal ketogenic foods contain less than 5g carbohydrates per 100g, which is a very low carb content. That does not mean you can't eat high-carb foods; it is a matter of working out what you are eating, the quantity and the carb count. For example, a 90% dark chocolate could contain 14g carbs per 100g, but you could consider eating just 1 or 2 squares as part of your daily carb count.

As a reminder for those who may have skipped the opening chapters, on the ketogenic way of eating, you ideally need to keep to around 20g total net carbohydrates per day. This may seem a little daunting, but it is surprising how easy this way of eating can be. Dairy, meat, eggs and fish are your staple foods, along with non-starchy vegetables. The joy of this way of eating is feeling satisfied after meals. Unlike a low-calorie or low-fat diet, you are not fighting hunger. Here are your staple foods:

Eggs

Meat, poultry and game

All types of meat are allowed, including:

- Offal

- Natural, cured meats *(such as bacon, pancetta and Parma ham)*

- Natural and cured sausages *(such as salami and chorizo).*
  Ensure all sausages are free from grains and as natural as possible.

Fish

Fish is a wonderful food. Choose oily fish such as salmon, tuna, mackerel, pilchards, haddock, trout etc. Almost all seafood is suitable, except swordfish and tilefish, which have a high mercury content.

Homemade broths

- Bone broth
- Chicken broth
- Vegetable broth

Dairy products

It is really important to always choose whole or full-fat dairy products. If you can, choose organic. Be aware of the carbohydrate count of dairy as lactose is a form of sugar. It can add up quite quickly, especially if you add milk to your cuppa. Some women may find dairy can hinder weight loss, especially those who are hormonal or pre-menopausal.

- Butter
- Full-fat cottage cheese
- Full-fat single, double and extra-thick cream
- Full-fat cream cheese
- Full-cream natural Greek yoghurt
- Whole (full-fat) milk
- All hard cheeses
- All soft cheeses
  (but not processed commercial cheese spreads such as Dairylea)

Oils and fats

The aim here is to eat healthy natural fats, that are stable and not inflammatory.

- Butter
- Coconut oil
- Duck/goose fat
- Ghee
- Lard
- Avocado oil
- Good-quality flax oil
- Good-quality olive oil
- Macadamia oil

Flavourings and condiments

All flavourings and condiments are okay, provided they do not contain sugars and preservatives or vegetable (seed) oils. Always read the label.

- Mayonnaise *(full-fat only; not from seeds oils)*
- Tomato ketchup *(homemade and sugar-free)*

Flours and thickeners

- Nut flours *(such as hazelnut, Brazil nut, walnut)*
- Seed flours *(such as flaxseed, sunflower)*

Almond flour	Ground almonds	Whey protein
Xanthan gum	Psyllium husk	Gelatine
Baking powder	Arrowroot	

Nuts and seeds

- Almonds (including almond flour and ground almonds)

Flaxseeds	Macadamia nuts	Pecans
Hazelnuts	Brazil nuts	Pine nuts
Pumpkin seeds	Sunflower seeds	Walnuts

- Coconut *(including coconut flours)*
- Pure nut butters *(but not peanut or cashew)*

PLEASE NOTE, THE FOLLOWING NUTS ARE HIGHER IN CARBS SO SHOULD BE AVOIDED

Cashews are one of the highest at 18.7g per 100g. Watch out for bags of mixed nuts, which may contain cashews.

Peanuts are a legume, so some people prefer to avoid them. Salted peanuts are on average around 6g per 100g.

Pistachios are almost 10g per 100g.

Chestnuts (kernel only) are 33.6g per 100g

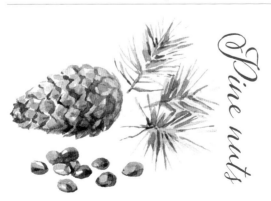

Pine nuts

Sweeteners

For more information see The Keto Store Cupboard (pages 16–25).

Vegetables

There is some confusion over vegetables. Most people say food grown above ground is low-carb and below ground is starchy and high-carb, but that is not strictly true. Celeriac is low-carb, as is swede, both of which are grown below ground. To avoid confusion, I have created two lists: the first made up of low-carb vegetables that equate to less than 5g per 100g. The second list comprises moderate carbs, with between 5g and 10g carbohydrates per 100g. Remember, you need to account for the volumes consumed. You would not eat 100g of ginger, so use your judgement.

Low-carb vegetables with less than 5g net carbohydrates per 100g *(raw weight)*

Asparagus	Aubergines	Bean sprouts
Broccoli	Brussel sprouts	Cabbage *(all varieties)*
Cauliflower	Celery	Chicory
Chillies	Courgettes	Cucumber
Celeriac	Endive	Fennel
Globe artichoke	Green beans	Jalapeño peppers
Jicama *(Mexican turnip)*	Kale	Leeks
Lettuce	Mushrooms	Olives
Pak choi	Peppers	Radishes
Rocket	Samphire	Sauerkraut
Spaghetti squash	Spinach	Spring onions
Suede	Sugar snap peas	Swiss chard
Shallots	Tomatoes	Turnip
Watercress		

Moderate-carb vegetables with between 5g and 10g net carbohydrates per 100g *(raw weight)*

Ginger 7.5g *(flesh)*	Beetroot 7.2g	Brown onions 6.4g
Butternut squash 7.9g	Carrots 6.8g	Pumpkin 6g
Red onion 7.4g	White onion 7.6g	

High-carb vegetables with net carbohydrates of over 10g per 100g *(raw weight)*

Parsnips 11.7g	Sweet potatoes 19.7g

Fruit

Most fruit is high in fructose and carbohydrates; however, the following are the lowest in carbohydrates in their raw state. Once again, think about the volume you are consuming. I use lemons a lot, but this is mainly the lemon zest which is virtually zero net carbohydrates per 100g, but a whole lemon shows around 6g per 100g. Note that rhubarb appears to come up anywhere between 0.7–5g per 100g depending on the source. I am not sure why there is such a discrepancy with data however for consistency, I am using my trusted computer-generated nutritional application which states 0.8g for raw stem flesh.

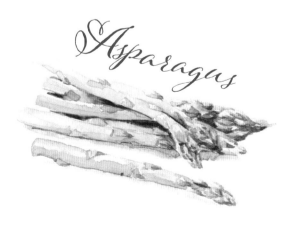

Asparagus

Low-carb fruits
(figures show net carbohydrates per 100g)

Avocados 1.9g *(flesh)*	Blackberries 5.1g	Blackcurrants 6.6g
Blueberries 9.1g	Cantaloupe melon 4.2g *(flesh only)*	Coconut flesh 6.2g
Cranberries 3.4g (fresh)	Gala melon 5.5g *(flesh only)*	Green olives 0.9g
Guavas 5.1g	Honeydew melon 6.7g *(flesh only)*	Kalamata olives 4.8g
Peaches 7.4g	Raspberries 4.6g	Rhubarb 0.8g *(raw stem flesh)*
Strawberries 6.1g	Watermelon 6.9g	

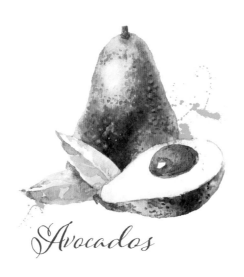

Avocados

High-carb fruits
(figures show net carbohydrates per 100g)

For occasional, moderate use only! Please be aware, it is very easy to overconsume these when you are trying to stick to 20g of total net carbohydrates per day.

Apples 9.9g	Apricots 7g	Bananas 20g
Cherries 11.5g (fresh)	Figs 9.5g (fresh)	Gooseberries 9.2g
Grapes 16.1g	Kiwi fruits 10.5g	
Mangoes 13.6g (flesh only)	Nectarines 8.7g	Oranges 8g
Oranges 8g	Papaya 8.7g	Peaches 7.4g
Pears 10.8 g	Pineapple 9.9g	Plums 8.7g

Chocolate

Should be dark – at least 85% cocoa solids – and you should always check the carbohydrate content. Unsweetened cocoa powder or cacao as well.

Herbs and spices

Unlimited herbs and spices but do read labels as a lot of spice blends can contain sugar and grain.

Drinks

Tea and coffee are fine as long as you are not affected by caffeine – watch the milk as the lactose can add up your carb count. Water and sparkling water are obviously fine too.

Foods you must not eat

This is a list of completely banned foods. Be sure to read all ingredients lists to ensure you are not inadvertently taking in any of the banned foods. This way of eating is all about eating 'real food', so you will find you will naturally avoid any processed or junk foods.

Baked goods
This includes cakes, biscuits, crackers and confectionary as all will contain grains and sugar. Anything made with flours from grains (wheat flour, cornflour, rye flour, barley flour, pea flour, rice flour) is also banned. Remember, all baked goods need to be made from scratch using low-carb, high-fat ingredients.

Bread
All forms of bread. Remember, you can make your own bread from scratch using keto ingredients.

All grains and corns
This includes wheat, oats, barley, rye, amaranth, quinoa, spelt, buckwheat, millet, cornflower, rice, couscous, teff, sorghum, brans, popcorn, polenta, corn thins and maize.

Beans (dried)
Such as lentils, chickpeas, red kidney beans, haricot beans and butterbeans.

Breaded and battered foods
For example, processed chicken nuggets, battered fish, breaded ham, etc.

Breakfast cereals
Avoid all breakfast cereals, even if the label states no added sugar. This includes muesli and granola.

Avoid all pastas, noodles and rice

This includes all forms of rice, including rice flours, as well as all pasta, including vegetable and gluten-free pasta.

Thickening agents

Avoid gravy powder, maize starch, cornflour or stock cubes as these contain grains and sugar. Opt instead for xanthan gum or coconut flour to thicken.

Drinks

- Beer, cider
- Fizzy drinks (sodas) of any description (although carbonated water can be drunk in moderate amounts)
- Lite, zero and diet drinks of any description
- Cordials

Dairy and dairy substitutes – please avoid any product that claims to be lite, low-fat or fat-free.

• Cheese spreads	• Commercial spreads	• Coffee creamers
• Commercial almond milk		
• Condensed milk	• Reduced-fat cow's milk	
• Rice milk	• Soya milk	• Ice cream

Seed and commercial oils

These oils and fats are very inflammatory and not stable. They are all processed, man-made and far from natural.

• Safflower	• Sunflower	• Canola
• Grapeseed	• Cottonseed	• Corn
• Hydrogenated or partially hydrogenated oils		
• Margarine	• Vegetable fats	

Chocolate

All commercial chocolate and confectionary (unless it contains at least 85% cocoa solids).

Commercial sauces, marinades and salad dressings

This includes all commercial sauces such as tomato ketchup, brown sauce and salad creams. Most salad dressings contain sugars and seed oils so it's best to make your own.

Fruits and vegetables

- Fruit juice of any kind
- Dried fruit
- Potatoes *(regular)*

Meat

- All unfermented soya *(vegetarian 'protein')*
- Meats cured with excessive amounts of sugar

General

- All fast food
- All low-fat foods
- All processed food
- Any food with added sugar such as glucose, dextrose, etc.

Sweeteners

- Agave anything
- Artificial sweeteners
  (aspartame, acesulfame K, saccharin, sucralose, Splenda)
- Dried fruit
- Fructose
- Fruit concentrates
- Grape juice
- Honey
- Malt
- Sugar
- Sugared or commercially pickled foods with sugar
- Sweets
- Syrups of any kind
  (with the exception of Sukrin Fibre Syrup made from erythritol)

List of recipes

Pantry Essentials

Index